PRAISE FOR *6-DAY BODY MAKEOVER*

"He is a true master of his craft . . . pragmatic, determined, and even dogged in his determination to succeed for his clients. His results never fail to astonish me."

—Jon A. Perlman, MD, FACS, clinical assistant professor
of plastic surgery at UCLA Medical Center

"Thurmond has developed a body type blueprinting system that allows readers to customize their diet regimen . . . Thurmond also gives fat-burning, low-intensity exercises to help lose weight and keep it off."

—*Toronto Star*

"A diet plan with staying power. [From dieter] Dolores Thompson, 'It worked for me! It's been six years and counting. I even became a personal trainer!'"

—*First for Women Magazine*

"A wealth of sound information."

—MonstersandCritics.com

"This book is packed with sensible tips and good advice . . . The book is written in a very accessible, easy-to-use style, with information presented in a clear, straightforward way."

—*Berkshire Eagle* (MA)

"Thurmond has menus and serving sizes all mapped out . . . sound weight reduction advice with quick and safe results."

—BookLoons.com

"Based on sound principles that just make sense about the body. Additionally, Michael gives you a 'what's next' after his 6-DAY BODY MAKE-OVER with valuable tips to get you going and keep you on target."

—Review-Books.com

MICHAEL THURMOND

6day
BODY
MAKEOVER

DROP ONE WHOLE DRESS OR PANT SIZE
IN <u>JUST</u> 6 DAYS—AND KEEP IT OFF

**WELLNESS
CENTRAL**

NEW YORK   BOSTON

Copyright © 2005 by Michael Thurmond and Provida Publishing, LLC
All rights reserved. Except as permitted under the U.S. Copyright Act of 1976, no part of this publication may be reproduced, distributed, or transmitted in any form or by any means, or stored in a database or retrieval system, without the prior written permission of the publisher.

Wellness Central
Hachette Book Group USA
237 Park Avenue, New York, NY 10017
Visit our Web site at www.HachetteBookGroupUSA.com

Wellness Central is an imprint of Grand Central Publishing.
The Wellness Central name and logo is a trademark of Hachette Book Group USA, Inc.

Printed in the United States of America

Originally published in hardcover
First Trade Edition: April 2006
10   9   8   7   6   5   4

The Library of Congress has cataloged the hardcover edition as follows:
Thurmond, Michael, personal trainer.
    6-day body makeover : drop one whole dress or pant size in just 6 days and keep it off / Michael Thurmond.—1st ed.
        p.   cm.
    Summary: "Michael Thurmond of television's 'Extreme Makeover' explains his scientific approach to eating, the 'blueprinting system,' which identifies a person's unique metabolism and body type and which foods will trigger the body to shed pounds" —Provided by the publisher.
    ISBN 0-446-57785-5
    1. Reducing diets.   2. Energy metabolism.   I. Title: Six-day body makeover.   II. Title.
    RM222.2.T489   2005
    613.2'5—dc22   2004027745

ISBN 978-0-446-69557-2 (pbk.)

This book is dedicated to my wonderful clients, to the millions of people who are using my make-over programs to transform their bodies and their health, and to you—the reader. May you take the information in this book, use it successfully, and pass it on to others. Continued health and success to all of you!

I would like to express my deep gratitude to the many people who were instrumental in making this book possible.

First, my heartfelt thanks and appreciation go to Jeff Clifford, Brady Caverly, and Lenny Sands, principals of Provida Life Sciences, who have played such a huge role in bringing my makeover programs to the attention of the world through three hit infomercials. Through skilled insight, creativity, and ingenuity, this Provida team took my basic approach to reshaping the human body and turned it into a phenomenal product called Michael Thurmond's *6-Week Body Makeover,* now one of the most popular and successful weight-loss and exercise programs around. Provida's work and proven ability at product development and marketing have been a springboard for me, but more than that have enabled millions of people to finally get in fabulous shape.

Dolores Thompson and Paul Duff, also of Provida Life Sciences, must also be acknowledged for their help in coordinating key aspects of this book, and most of all for helping to inspire the millions of people who have learned how to make over their bodies using my techniques.

I would also like to thank Barbara Lowenstein, who must be one of the greatest agents anywhere, for seeing the value of this book and bringing it to light. My thanks also go to Maggie Greenwood-Robinson, PhD, whose talents, experience, creativity, and professionalism were invaluable to this project. The staff at Warner Books, particularly Diana Baroni, have been enthusiastic from the start, and I greatly appreciate their assistance and coordination with every aspect of this book.

I gratefully thank Benita Heet, who manages my company, Body Makeover Systems, with incredible efficiency, and who schedules me, centers me, and enriches my life. I could do nothing without my wonderful staff, whose help and support made this book possible.

Finally, I would like to thank all my wonderful clients who have trusted me to guide them through their body transformations.

Contents

Introduction   *You Can Be Slimmer by Friday*   *xi*

chapter **1**

Blueprinting: Discover How Your Individual
Metabolism Reacts to Food 1

chapter **2**

Why It Works: The Metabolic Principles Behind the
6-Day Body Makeover 21

chapter **3**

The *6-Day Body Makeover* Basics 41

chapter **4**

Customized Eating Plans That Guarantee Rapid Results:
The *6-Day Body Makeover* Meals and Menus 49

chapter **5**

**Staying on Track: Simple Secrets That Make
It Easy and Foolproof** 109

chapter **6**

**Your Fat-Burning Weapon: Long Slow
Distance Exercise** 127

chapter **7**

***6-Day Body Makeover* Tips from A to Z** 145

chapter **8**

**The Seventh Day and Beyond:
What to Do Next** 163

appendix A

The *6-Day Body Makeover* Recipes 183

appendix B

Customizations for Special Medical Conditions 223

appendix C

Additional Resources 233

You Can *Be Slimmer by Friday*

Suppose today is Sunday. Imagine gazing in the mirror next Friday—just six days from now—and seeing yourself leaner, lighter, and fitting into a dress, jeans, pants, or some other outfit that is one size smaller than you normally wear. There you are, ready for the weekend: You are slimmer. Your tummy is flatter. You look better than you have in a very long time.

Wouldn't it be terrific if that image in the mirror could become reality for you? Well, it can, and it will. And you won't have to starve yourself down to size. Or punish yourself with unending reps, sets, laps, and other sweaty, exhausting forms of exercise.

Welcome to my *6-Day Body Makeover,* a one-of-a-kind plan that is completely customized to your own body type and metabolism, and designed to accelerate your weight loss so that you see dramatic results—quickly. How quickly? In just six days. You can lose up to a pound each day, or more, depending on how much you weigh to begin with, plus trim off flabby inches from your body. What you'll experience will be so motivating and so simple that you will want to continue your weight loss beyond those six days, right on toward your goal weight, because you look and feel so fabulous.

There's more: To achieve your goal weight, you can apply the very same principles of this program, modified for longer-term weight loss, and ultimately get to your goal.

You'll find out how to transition from the *6-Day Body Makeover* to a program that will help you keep going toward your ideal size. What's more, you can stay at that size by putting into practice the keep-it-off guidelines you'll learn here. Once you lose all the pounds you want to lose, you'll want to stick to your new eating and exercise habits because you will look and feel so terrific. In fact, those new stay-in-shape habits will become your normal way of life.

How can I be so sure?

Because over the past two decades, I've worked with thousands of people, from every walk of life—people just like you—to help them transform their bodies into a shape they once only dreamed about. They turned their dream bodies into reality by using a diet designed just for them to totally make over their bodies in a very short time, melting away as much as 10 (or sometimes more) pounds in just under a week, then going on from there to shed even more weight. And you can do it, too. I'm very excited for you because you're going to see over the next six days such a dramatic change in what your body looks like and feels like that everyone you know will keep asking for your secret.

That "secret," found in this book, is an accelerated version of my *6-Week Body Makeover*, a program that I've developed over the past 20 years that allows you to eat more and exercise less, yet still lose weight and reshape your body, all in as little as six weeks. It's a comprehensive program that includes targeted body-sculpting routines that you can follow if you need to lose more weight. Later in the book, I'll give you more information on how to get started on that program. For now, let's get focused on the *next six days*.

When I set out to design the *6-Day Body Makeover*, I wanted to fill a huge void in the weight-loss market. Thousands and thousands of "diets" are available telling you how to lose weight, but most of them are usually difficult to stick to because it takes too long to succeed, and these diets typically involve deprivation. So when faced with any temptation, whether it's an ice cream sundae or a bag of chips, most dieters throw in the towel, get discouraged, and feel like they can never succeed on any type of diet. Until the *6-Day Body Makeover*, there really hasn't been a practical program for rapid, short-term weight loss that allows you to lose a lot of weight in a short time, and do it safely, without deprivation.

Working directly with thousands of people over the years gave me the unique opportunity to listen to what they most desired in a weight-loss program. And what they wanted was to see results fast—so that they could lose weight quickly and keep it off. People were constantly asking me, "How can I get in shape for my daughter's wedding . . . for a pool party next weekend . . . for an important date . . . to fit into a dress that's now too snug?" They'd tell me, "I don't have time to lose weight. I've only got a week! It's too late to start a diet!" Desperate questions and comments such as these made me realize that millions of people could benefit from a simple, practical program that would take off pounds and inches in a very short time—just six days—and drop one whole dress or pant size. Yes, there's a need in this country to shed multiple pounds to help eradicate the alarming rise in obesity in this country. And this program will help jump-start your metabolism so you can begin this journey. The *6-Day Body Makeover* is the tool that will help people like you begin to see positive changes in your weight in just under a week—and teach you to maintain those positive changes. That's why I decided to create this program. My clients who have used the *6-Day Body Makeover* are amazed at how quickly they see results, and it gives them the confidence to go on to lose even more weight if they need to. This is a simple, doable program, with a refreshing and unique promise: dropping a whole dress or pant size in six days. And I know you can do it.

"Am I happy with the results? Ecstatic! I look years younger; I'm full of energy and thinner than I ever dreamed possible."

—Linda W.

Okay, ready, set . . . put your thumb in the waistband of your jeans or skirt. Could you use a little more room there? Do you want to fit into a smaller size? Or do you have a party or a big date this weekend that you want to look your best for? How about an upcoming class reunion or a family gathering? Wouldn't you like to fit into that new outfit you just bought in order to make a great first impression? Do you need to fit into a wedding dress, a cocktail dress, or a tux? Do you wish you could drop those stubborn, final pounds and get closer to your goal weight? Wouldn't you like to shed unwanted weight that you gained over a holiday or vacation?

The *6-Day Body Makeover* is a surefire way to get that weight off very quickly—and do it with maintainable results. It's a very practical tool for achieving any of the above goals. The story of Margaret, one of my makeover clients who used this tool, is typical.

Margaret had a closet full of two sizes of clothes—what she considered her "fat" clothes (size 16s) and her "thin" clothes (size 10s). Using one of my makeover programs, Margaret lost 32 pounds in six weeks and was able to fit in size 10 dresses. But to hit to her desired weight of 135, she had to break through a plateau. Margaret had been in a holding pattern above 140 pounds for a couple of weeks. Frustrated by her inability to reach her goal, she wanted to smash her scale into smithereens because the pounds wouldn't budge. I suggested that she try the *6-Day Body Makeover* in order to get the needle on her scale out of the "stuck" position. She agreed to give it a whirl. After completing the six-day program, Margaret lost 6 pounds. She was looking better than ever and feeling more energetic than ever. She fit beautifully into a size 10 and looked gorgeous in her new clothes. (Incidentally, I told her to rid her closet of those "fat" clothes so that she would no longer have reminders of herself as a "fat person," or think of herself in that self-defeating way.)

Here's what Sally, another makeover client, told me recently: "I love the *6-Day Body Makeover*! Last summer, I used it to get in shape for my son's wedding. I lost 9 pounds and 11½ inches that week. The program took me from a size 18 to a size 16."

Sally continued to use my makeover techniques to lose additional weight, ultimately reaching her goal of wearing a size 8. At one point, she gained several pounds over the Easter holiday. This discouraging experience motivated her to use the *6-Day Body Makeover* again. To her surprise, she lost 8 pounds in just six days. "I never would have believed I could lose that much weight, so quickly. The *6-Day Body Makeover* has made all the difference. It's just a part of my life now." Even today, Sally still uses the program to manage her weight and stay at a size in which she looks and feels her best.

Nancy also represents the type of client who knows how valuable the *6-Day Body Makeover* can be. Listen to what she told me: "This program has changed my life and prepared me for one of the most important days of my life, my wedding! I've success-fully used the *6-Day Body Makeover* several times. It is amazing and really works! I use it when I feel like I've added a few pounds and want to get them off quickly; when I'm on a plateau, it seems to shake things up and start the weight loss again. I've lost any-where from 4 to 6 pounds in the six days and easily an inch or more on my waist. I've recently gained back over 10 pounds since my wedding, and I'm planning a *6-Day Body Makeover* next week! I'm sure it will be just what I need to get back on track."

As you and I go through this book together over the next six days, you'll learn in greater detail how you can make the *6-Day Body Makeover* part of your life, too. Once you discover how you can lose pounds and inches and drop an entire size in just six days—and once you learn how easy this is to do—you, too, will become a believer.

For now, I understand how frustrated you've probably been with your efforts because you've gotten nowhere. Why even put in the effort if you're not going to see results? I always say, "Don't go to work unless you're going to receive a good paycheck." Like that paycheck, you need a reward, and you'll get lots of rewards with this program! This time will be different. This time you'll lose fat, trim inches, eat foods that love your body, and recharge your self-esteem. You'll feel good, you'll be energized, and you'll be in a positive frame of mind.

If you follow the exact instructions outlined in this book, in just six short days you'll lose enough weight to fit into clothes that are one whole size smaller than you are wear-ing at this very instant. There are no gimmicks, because the program is based on basic, sound science. It isn't one of those diets where you eat nothing but cottage cheese and grapefruit. This isn't one of those programs where you have to mix up foul-tasting pow-dered drinks or take pills. On this program, you eat nothing but delicious natural foods. In fact, this plan uses food as a tool to burn fat.

The *6-Day Body Makeover* approaches the goal of weight loss from an entirely dif-ferent perspective than the low-calorie model or the low-carb model. You eat, and eat a lot—and drop pounds without feeling deprived or having to count calories. In fact, for the *6-Day Body Makeover* to work, you must eat frequently in order to speed up your metabolism to the point that it burns calories faster. Eating constantly and eating all the required food on the plan are very important to your success. This plan is designed to produce quick results—and let's be honest, that's what you want—not because it starves you down to size but because its carefully designed balance of food adjusts your body metabolically so that you burn fat, day in and day out. You'll probably eat more than you've ever eaten on any other diet before in your life. Because the key to this program is just that: eating. You'll eat five to six times a day and you'll still lose weight, steadily and efficiently. This is just the kind of reward that can turn these next six days into a life-long desire to achieve and maintain a beautiful body.

There's no carb counting on this program, either. When you follow the eating plan that is tailored for you, you automatically consume the correct amount and type of carbohydrates for your metabolism. You do not want to cut carbs from your diet, since this practice is extremely self-defeating. If you cut out the carbs, at some point your body will go into what is known as a catabolic state—it begins consuming its own muscle tissue for energy. You need muscle tissue for body shape and to support an active, fat-burning metabolism. Carbohydrates supply the bodily energy to support the growth and repair of muscle tissue, as well as the fuel to support brain function. You cannot build and maintain lean, toned muscle without carbohydrates. And you need muscle for curves, definition, tone, and overall shape.

There's another crucial problem with low-carb diets: They deprive your brain of its favorite fuel source: carbs! Brain cells need glucose from the breakdown of carbs to function; it is the fuel your brain normally uses. In absence of glucose, you can feel spacey, unable to think or perform correctly at work, at school, or anywhere. Plus, it can cause you to be moody, and even unmotivated to achieve your weight-loss goals. Fad-dish low-carbohydrate diets are unhealthy and damaging to your body, mind, and spirit.

And if you're hypoglycemic (low blood sugar), which is relatively common in our society, you really don't want to cut out carbohydrates, because carbs help keep your blood sugar at an even level. You shouldn't go on a low-carbohydrate diet of any type if you expect to look and feel your best.

With this book, I'll take you through easy-to-follow, step-by-step guidelines on what you can do to succeed. Essentially, this plan provides customized menu plans that can help you drop inches and pounds fast. Through my exclusive Body Type Blueprinting system, you'll determine your body type, how your body reacts to food, and how your metabolism is programmed to process the foods you eat. Some people can eat foods such as pasta or bread and not gain an ounce of weight. With others, it seems all they have to do is think about processed carbohydrates, and they pack on the pounds. That's because everyone's metabolism is different. Your best friend may be able to burn up bowls of pasta, while you do better by staying away from it. Because of these metabolic differences, everyone must select the specific types of food to work with their individual metabolism. You have to take into account your body's own chemistry and know which foods work best for you. Once you have this information, you can stop the frustrating cycle of going on and off diets that don't work. When you eat foods especially selected for your body chemistry, while eating more meals each day, you experience the rapid weight loss you are hoping for. My unique Blueprinting system will help you identify your specific body type and identify the *right* foods to spark weight loss for you. Blueprinting is what makes this program work, and it is what other weight-loss programs lack.

The *6-Day Body Makeover* will also introduce you to a totally different approach to cardiovascular exercise that will accelerate your fat loss, but without the drudgery of high-intensity workouts. By moving your body at an acceptable pace and using a special form of breathing known as Abdominal Breathing to oxygenate your body, you'll become trimmer and more fit, plus feel more energetic and invigorated than you have in years.

As long as you eat according to your Blueprint, this customized strategy of eating fat-burning foods—and lots of them—along with my unconventional approach to cardiovascular exercise will result in dramatic, quick weight loss in just six short days.

There's more. This approach to eating can help you feel and look younger. It's no secret that eating the right kinds of foods does have an anti-aging effect. Eating fish, for example, improves

"After the holidays, I gained 7 pounds, and all my clothes were starting to fit too tightly. Nothing really looked good on me anymore. Determined to shed that holiday weight, I tried the 6-Day Body Makeover, *and by the end of the six days, all the holiday weight vanished. I returned to a weight at which I feel comfortable and look much better. I never felt like I was crash dieting because there was so much food to eat, and the program was easy to follow."*

—*Marcia S.*

the tone and texture of your skin and slows down the aging process, due to this food's protein and fat balance. A diet rich in fruits and vegetables, like you'll eat on this program, supplies antioxidants, too. The eating plan you'll follow on the *6-Day Body Makeover* helps replace these anti-aging nutrients. You'll be drinking plenty of water on this program, too. Apart from being essential for life, water helps you achieve a better complexion by making your skin look plump and practically wrinkle-free. So you see: The healthy foods you'll be eating over the next six days—and hopefully, for the rest of your life—will boost your body and your health. Food is really the best makeover tool there is!

Let me emphasize too that none of my makeover programs was created by accident, but rather through years of research and experimentation. Their genesis really began when I was growing up in Los Angeles, California. Remember the fattest kid in school? Well, that was me. In fact, I was overweight as far back as I can remember, and that is a very painful way to grow up. On top of being fat, I was uncoordinated and unathletic. In school, kids constantly teased and tormented me, and when it was time to choose teams in gym class, I was always picked last.

Whenever I looked in the mirror, I hated my flabby, awkward body. I felt that I wasn't as good as anyone else, and I had no self-confidence. Even so, I would daydream about what it would be like to have large, chiseled muscles, a washboard stomach, and a thin waist. But I didn't know how to make that dream come true.

By the time I was 11, I was clinically obese, so my parents put me on a medically supervised diet that included mild doses of Dexedrine, better known as uppers. That approach didn't work, nor did other countless diets that I went on. I had practically given up on life—and I was just a kid!

As a teenager I learned to lift weights. I didn't lose weight; I just got stronger. I still had no idea how to change the shape of my body in order to achieve the physique I had always dreamed of. That all changed when I was 17 and found myself stationed on an aircraft carrier on the way to the Gulf of Tonkin in Vietnam. It was there that I met a shipmate from Brooklyn who was a bodybuilder, affectionately nicknamed Bugsy. Training with Bugsy taught me how to use weights to sculpt and shape my body. It was an entirely new way of exercising contrary to everything I had ever done. I discovered that working harder wasn't necessarily better and that changing the shape of my body was relatively easy once I knew what I was doing. This discovery would lead to the development of my Precision Sculpting System, one of the components of my *6-Week Body Makeover* program.

Still, something was missing—and that "something" was food and how the body processes it. After being assigned to kitchen duty in the mess hall, I had the opportunity to experiment with my diet. Over the next several months, I learned how food worked in my body—which foods made me gain body fat and which foods made me lose it. Once I started eating the right foods for my metabolism, the fat pounds started melting off my body.

Over the next 10 years, I continued to research and experiment in order to refine my program. I scoured all the information I could find on biology, physiology, and chemistry—any science that would give me insights into how my body reacted to food and responded to exercise. Soon I had refined my program to the point that I had the power to make my body change in any way I wanted. This led me to competitive bodybuilding where the ability to change, shape, and sculpt my physique gave me a tremendous advantage, and I won numerous titles. I felt like I was in control of my body for the first time in my life.

Soon others began asking me to help them make over their bodies. I started with a couple of overweight teens in my neighborhood and worked closely with them so that they would never have to go through the same suffering and pain that I had endured as a child. I taught them how to eat and to sculpt their bodies in my small home gym. Their bodies began to change—and change

> *"I was never hungry. The way the food plan is put together makes you lose weight, because you're eating foods that work with your metabolism. I ate all day long. My metabolism really responded to that, and I started dropping a pound a day."*
>
> —*Jim F.*

dramatically. Other teens filtered in, and I taught them how to use food to lose fat, how to employ simple cardiovascular exercise to accelerate fat loss, and how to use weight training to sculpt their bodies.

The results these kids achieved were phenomenal, and pretty soon their parents, relatives, and other adults wanted the secret to having a beautiful body. So I began training adults in my makeover approach. Word of mouth traveled to the entertainment industry, and before long actors, actresses, and models, desperate to make over their bodies for new roles and photo shoots, came calling. By 1985, I had codified my makeover methods into what is now known as the *6-Week Body Makeover*. Today, my company, Body Makeovers, Inc., employs more than 100 trainers, each one personally schooled in my makeover methods and techniques. These are the very same methods and techniques I use with people selected to appear on ABC's hit show *Extreme Makeovers*. As a member of the show's "Extreme Team," I help these people lose weight quickly prior to, and after, having plastic surgery, plus help them add lean, curvaceous muscle to their physiques and sculpt their bodies before and after surgery.

One of the results of these many years of experience, exhaustive research, experimentation, and trial and error is the *6-Day Body Makeover* program you have in your hands. On this program, you will be surprised and delighted by how fast the results come when you use food to lose fat. When you do that, your body has no choice but to drop pounds, and drop them fast. If you start your makeover on a Sunday, by the time Friday arrives—the start of a new weekend—you will see a significant difference in the way you look and feel. You *can* be slimmer by Friday.

The proof that these makeover techniques work is in the measurable success, in both pounds and inches lost, that we see in our clients.

I know the testimonials you'll read throughout this book sound miraculous, like something that should be filed away in the "too-good-to-be-true" department, but they are all true. And you can experience similar results. Your body will start changing the first six days. Transforming your body really isn't as hard as you think it is once you learn the right information. You're holding that information in your hands right now, and with it you can start giving your body a new lease on life. So let's get started. Let's take the first step toward making you a whole dress or pant size smaller in just six days.

CHAPTER 1

Blueprinting: Discover How Your Individual Metabolism Reacts to Food

Have you ever wondered why your rail-thin friend can eat ice cream, bread, french fries, and other types of foods and not gain an ounce—and why you, on the other hand, seem to put on pounds just looking at that stuff? Could it be that your metabolism has downshifted to neutral or perhaps stalled altogether?

If you even suspect that your metabolism is puttering along, you're probably correct. But you don't dare suggest it, since many weight-control experts regard "it's my metabolism" as a lame cover-up for the steady diet of pizza and ice cream they're sure you've been on. The truth, however, is that your metabolism may really be out of whack, so the fact that you're prone to weight gain may not be entirely your fault. Don't despair: You're not doomed to a life of plus sizes and seat belt extenders. You can recharge your metabolism by eating and exercising in ways that are completely customized to your individual metabolic needs.

You see: The first key to losing weight *quickly* is determining how your body responds to different types of food. Not all metabolisms are created equal. Everyone is different. Not everyone can eat exactly the same foods the same way and get the same results. Foods that help one person stay lean may have no impact on another person, and someone else may gain weight eating those same foods. That's why your friend's metabolism burns up those surplus calories as heat, while yours stores them as fat. To be successful at weight control, you must discover how your own metabolism reacts to food: what foods work for you to help you lose weight, and what foods don't. You must customize your diet to your own unique metabolism and biochemistry. Once you do that, you can eat more, not less, and ultimately have the body you want.

The reason you can achieve that goal, plus lose one whole size in six days, is because this program is tailored precisely to you. It is not a one-size-fits-all plan, because one size does not fit all when it comes to nutrition and dieting. You'll need to customize your diet by using my Body Type Blueprinting system, which is explained later in this chapter. It begins with a written questionnaire, with corresponding illustrations, that accurately and easily pinpoints your body type and metabolism. This Blueprint will help determine which of five standard metabolisms you have and which of five standard body types best fits you. By completing the questionnaire, you'll identify your body type and you'll learn, once and for all, how your metabolism ticks. After all, you can't get it running in high gear until you know how to shift it there.

Once you do your Blueprint and understand how your metabolism works, you can start eating *more* of the foods that cause you to lose weight and keep your body functioning at the healthiest possible level. When that happens, weight loss becomes automatic, because you've created a chemical reaction in your body with predictable results: a smaller dress or pant size in just six days. If you stick to this six-day program, it can work for you virtually 100 percent of the time—and you'll jump-start your metabolism so that your body becomes more efficient at burning food as fuel rather than storing it as fat.

Your Metabolic Machinery

There is a lot to this business of metabolism. Derived from a Greek word meaning "change," *metabolism* is the sum of all the chemical changes and reactions that happen inside your body. Some of these reactions serve to build up various substances such as muscle, fat, bone, hair, or nails. Other reactions serve to break down food, fat, or glycogen (a form of carbohydrate stored in muscles) for energy. Both the building up (called anabolic) and the breaking down (called catabolic) are going on simultaneously, every second of the day. The main raw material—the stuff your body uses for metabolism—is food, or more accurately the nutrients in food.

The speed at which your body does all of its metabolic tasks is referred to as metabolic rate, and it eventually regulates how much you weigh on the scale. If you have a very fast metabolism, your body can easily burn all the calories you take in. That's why some people can regularly eat a pint of ice cream and not put on weight. Their metabolisms are so fast, anything they eat is rapidly converted to fuel. On the other hand, if you have a slow metabolism, even a spoonful of ice cream goes straight to your hips, because your body can't burn up all the calories you feed it, and many of them get deposited as fat. Yours may be a *fat-storing* metabolism when what you want is a *fat-burning* metabolism.

I often use the analogy of a bonfire to explain how the body's metabolism works and to help people understand how to manipulate their diets to burn body fat. So try to imagine your metabolism as a bonfire, and the food you eat as logs you put on the fire. If the bonfire is burning big and hot, it has no trouble consuming the additional wood you put on it. You put on a giant log, and it burns in minutes. To keep the bonfire going, though, you have to keep feeding it with pieces of wood, or else it will die out. Unless you keep throwing wood on the fire, the blaze will turn into a pile of embers. Your metabolism works the same way: If you continue to feed it with the right foods in the right amounts at the right intervals, you stoke your metabolism. It will run very efficiently, and your body will burn that food for fuel. When you have a very fast metabolism, your body can easily burn whatever you feed it.

Conversely, if the bonfire begins to die out and burn more slowly, it doesn't burn as quickly the new wood you put on it. If you put a big log on the smoldering embers of a fire, the log is liable just to sit there. It may take all night for it to slowly burn away. Again, your metabolism works the same way. When your metabolism is very slow, it can't burn all the calories you feed it. The food you eat just sits there and eventually gets stored as fat. Put another way: A slow metabolism is not burning food for fuel; it is storing food as body fat.

Let's go back to the bonfire for a moment. Suppose you toss a few old newspapers into the fire. What happens? Poof! The flames shoot up fast in response. The newspapers incinerate in milliseconds and disappear—but so does the intensity of the flames. The fire dies as fast as it was ignited. Those newspapers are like foods high in sugar and simple, processed carbohydrates. They burn up fast, but don't do much to fan the flames of your metabolic fire. In fact, they slow it down. You need clean, solid-burning fuel just like the bonfire needs a good solid log. That's where the proper food comes in—clean slow-burning food like lean proteins and wholesome, natural carbohydrates. These foods can help fan the flames of a sluggish metabolism, and you'll be eating them on the *6-Day Body Makeover*.

Now that you have the picture of how metabolism works, let's talk specifically about you. What factors affect your metabolic rate?

Age

Remember when you were a kid and could eat anything you wanted and not gain much weight? But after you had your first child or turned 40, the pounds started sneaking on, and now it seems harder than ever to keep that weight off. It's true that metabolic rate slows down the older we get. But there's good news and bad news here. First, the bad news: Part of this decline is due to age-related losses of muscle tissue. The good news is that you can reverse, or even halt, this process if you lift weights as part of your exercise program and build metabolism-boosting muscle tissue in the process.

There's more good news: In addition to exercise, the foods you choose on this program—which will be the right fuel mixture for your metabolism—will effectively manipulate your metabolic rate so that you can regain the body of your youth, or the body of your dreams.

Gender

Comparatively, men have faster metabolisms than women do—between 10 and 20 percent faster, in fact. One of the main reasons for this is that men have more muscle and less fat than women do, and muscle uses more energy than fat tissue (which is metabolically inactive). But anyone, male or female, can add muscle to the body through weight training and other forms of exercise, supported by a metabolism-enhancing diet. If you build muscle, you'll raise your metabolic rate and burn off more fat, even at rest.

Perhaps you've recently joined a gym and/or started an exercise program, or you've tried some form of exercise in the past. More than likely, you have been disappointed by your failure to lose weight with exercise and are wondering why. The reason is that weight loss will not happen without the right eating plan. Nutrition and exercise work hand in hand to achieve the best results.

Physical Activity Level

Anything that gets your heart pumping and your muscles moving—whether it's jogging or weight training—will stimulate your metabolism so that you'll burn energy at a faster rate than usual for as long as 24 hours after you perform the exercise, in addition to the immediate burn-off accomplished during the activity. Exercise, particularly weight training, does something else, too: It reduces the body fat you're carrying and increases your muscle mass. If you have a high ratio of muscle to body fat, you'll have a higher metabolic rate. That means you can eat more and not gain weight, because you can burn more. Muscle is like a furnace that never goes off. It constantly burns food for fuel at a rapid rate, every moment of the day, even when you're asleep.

One more important point: Exercise must be done correctly to maximize your body's ability to burn fat—and that doesn't necessarily mean working out hard. In fact, hard workouts often have the exact wrong effect, as you will learn in chapter 6.

Genetics

Your ability to fit into your jeans is partially affected by your genes, a set of instructions that tells your cells what to do. You can inherit genes that regulate whether you have a fast metabolism or a slow one. If you've had trouble losing or controlling your weight your entire life, then you were probably born with a slow metabolism. Your body type was inherited, too, just like the color of your hair, the shape of your nose, or your mother's hips. The tendency to store fat, particularly in certain parts of the body, is also inherited.

Fortunately, genetics are not the biggest factor in metabolism and can be easily overcome when you customize your diet and exercise to your unique body type. That is what you'll begin to do in this chapter with my Blueprinting process: determine what kind of metabolism you were born with, or have developed, so you can select the right foods and cardiovascular exercise to accelerate it—and begin burning fat immediately.

Food and Diet

The number one factor influencing your metabolic rate is what you eat. Unfortunately, many of the staples in our diets these days have the ability to slow down our metabolic machinery. Foods laced with lots of simple sugars, such as soda, candy, baked goods, fruit juice, and other sweets, as well as many processed foods like breads and pastas, particularly when consumed in the wrong combination with other foods, will release a hormone that essentially tells your body to stop converting food to energy and start forming body fat instead. That hormone is insulin, and although it has a number of useful functions in your body, an excess of sugar-laden foods causes insulin to go haywire and wreak metabolic havoc in your system. As you can imagine, once that happens you are virtually doomed to gain weight, particularly if your metabolism is already sluggish from the factors discussed above. Much of my program is concerned with controlling the levels of sugar and insulin in your bloodstream to keep them from telling your body to form fat.

The foods you will select on this program are metabolism-maximizing foods. They can fan the flames of a sluggish metabolism, and they do this by generating a postmeal blaze inside your body. Digesting food is a calorie-burning activity (as is exercise). After you eat a meal, your body works hard to convert what you've eaten into energy. A portion of this food energy is given off as heat—which is referred to as the thermic effect of food. The more food you burn off as heat, the less you store. Some foods have a higher thermic effect than others, which means they are better choices for boosting your metabolism. Nearly 30 percent of the calories from protein, for example, and approximately 15 percent of the calories from carbohydrates are burned off as heat during digestion, whereas calories from dietary fat are more readily stored as fat by the body.

Restrictive crash-type dieting doesn't help your metabolism, either. When you go on one of these diets, your metabolism regards even a moderate calorie cutback as a signal that starvation is at hand, and your body starts packing away fat in case this "famine" goes on indefinitely. Even though you're eating less food, your body starts metabolizing it more slowly—burning less for energy and storing more as fat as a survival mechanism. This means you may not lose weight. In fact, it is very possible to go on a crash diet and actually *gain* weight because your body goes into starvation mode and starts hoarding body fat as storage fuel for survival. What's more, crash diets often slow that metabolism because you're not eating enough food to keep your metabolic fire stoked. That's why most people, after failing on a diet, often gain more weight back than they lost. They've slowed their metabolism so much that virtually everything they eat gets stored as fat. Restrictive diets slow your metabolism, and they can make you fat.

If you look back through this list of factors influencing your metabolism, it's obvious that the two you can control are your diet and your physical activity. That's incredibly powerful news, if you think about it, because both factors are totally within your control. You have the power to change your metabolism from slow to fast, and in the process get a lean, healthy body as quickly as possible.

As our first step in that direction, you and I must identify your own individual metabolism and body type using my Body Type Blueprinting system. It will give you information on how your body works so that you select foods that trigger weight loss and avoid foods that cause you to gain. Grab a pen or pencil, and let's get started.

Blueprinting Questionnaire: What's Your Body Type?

Body type is a method of describing the percentage of fat to muscle on your frame, your bone structure, your overall proportions, and your metabolism, since there is a correlation between body type and how efficiently your body metabolizes food for fuel. There are five different body types, each based on solid science, and one of them will fit you. This questionnaire is a very easy method for identifying your body type and learning how your individual metabolism functions. It takes approximately 5 to 10 minutes to answer all 48 questions and complete the scoring. Read each statement carefully and circle only those statements that best describe you right now. Be as honest as you can; there are no right or wrong answers. Take your time and do not rush through this questionnaire.

Once you're finished with the questionnaire, you'll know which of five body types you have. Then you'll be ready to move directly into the next chapters, where you'll learn which foods are compatible with your metabolism and the diet that is right for you. That means you'll be able to start losing weight right away and looking better than you have in a long time.

Check the box beside each comment that most accurately describes you. Remember, be honest in your answers.

- ❑ 1. When I gain weight, it's all over my entire body.

- ❑ 2. I have always been athletic, but recently the pounds have begun to creep up.

- ❑ 3. There was a time, after I graduated from high school, when I could eat practically anything I wanted and never gain an ounce.

- ❑ 4. It seems like no matter how little I eat, I gain weight.

- ❑ 5. For as long as I can remember, all I had to do was look at food and I would gain weight.

- ❑ 6. If I am even an hour late for a regular meal, I get ravenously hungry.

- ❑ 7. Even if I lost all the fat I wanted, I'd never be a skinny model type. I have more meat on my bones than that.

- ❑ 8. I have lots of energy. People are always amazed at how much I get done in a day.

- ❑ 9. Most of the time I can hide my weight in my clothes, but I wouldn't consider being seen in a swimsuit.

- ❑ 10. I am rarely hungry at mealtime.

- ❑ 11. Obesity runs in my family (many close members of my family are 50 pounds or more overweight).

- ❑ 12. I get hungry very soon after I eat.

- ❑ 13. If all the fat on my body disappeared, I think I would look great.

❑ 14. If all the fat on my body disappeared, I think I might be skinny or bony.

15. To get my ideal body, I will have to lose:
   ❑ Women: one to two dress sizes (for instance, from size 8 to 6 or 4).
   ❑ Men: 2 to 4 inches on my waist.

16. To get my ideal body, I will have to lose:
   ❑ Women: three to four dress sizes (for instance, from size 14 to 8 or 6).
   ❑ Men: 4 to 8 inches on my waist.

17. To get my ideal body, I will have to lose:
   ❑ Women: five or more dress sizes (from size 18 to 8 or 6, for example).
   ❑ Men: 8 or more inches on my waist.

❑ 18. If I go more than two or three hours without eating, I get shaky or irritable.

❑ 19. There are parts of my body that are too muscular (my butt or thighs or my arms).

❑ 20. At the same time that I lose weight, I would like to increase the size of some of my muscles to give my body shape and definition.

❑ 21. It is only as I got older or had children that I started to have trouble with my weight.

❑ 22. I have very low energy levels much of the time.

❑ 23. I worry that I am so overweight, it is jeopardizing my health.

❑ 24. If I go a long time without eating, I get a feeling of panic.

❑ 25. As far as I can remember, I have never been so thin that people would call me "bony" or "skinny."

❑ 26. Parts of my body are too thin (skinny arms, thighs, or calves).

❑ 27. When I get more physical activity in my life, my body loses fat fairly quickly.

28. I need to lose weight *all* over my body.

29. Because of my weight, it is very hard for me to do any kind of exercise.

30. If I don't eat on schedule, I simply can't control what I eat at the next meal.

31. Even though I may have more fat than I want, the body underneath is still pretty solid (hard or firm underneath when I flex my muscle).

32. At some point in my adult life, people have said to me, "You should gain weight; you look too thin."

33. There are parts of my body that are *not* overweight.

34. I currently eat only twice a day.

35. I have had serious weight problems for nearly my entire life.

36. Sometimes when I get up too quickly, I feel light-headed or dizzy.

37. If I had to describe myself as physically either "strong" or "weak," I would tend to say "strong."

38. If I had to describe myself as physically either "strong" or "weak," I would tend to say "weak."

39. I tend to gain weight in specific areas (belly, love handles, thighs) while much of the rest of my body stays normal.

40. I have been off and on diets for much of my adult life.

41. I believe that I am genetically doomed to be fat and will always be fat.

42. After exercise, I often feel like I am starving.

43. If I flex my arm, I can feel a muscle.

44. More than being overweight, my problem is that my body lacks shape or definition.

45. I have only had trouble with my weight for the last three to five years.

❑ 46. I used to be very athletic, but I don't even recognize my body anymore.

❑ 47. If I had to pick a shape to describe my body, it would probably be "round."

❑ 48. If I am tense or anxious, eating a candy bar, bread, or pasta tends to calm me down.

SCORING AND INTERPRETATION

Next, follow these steps to total your answers and identify your unique body type.

STEP 1. Circle the number below of each corresponding question you checked in the questionnaire. For example, if you checked number 11 in the questionnaire, you would circle number 11 in column 5.

1	2	3	4	5	6
1	2	3	4	5	6
7	8	9	10	11	12
13	14	15	16	17	18
19	20	21	22	23	24
25	26	27	28	29	30
31	32	33	34	35	36
37	38	39	40	41	42
43	44	45	46	47	48

Total the number of circles in each column.

STEP 2. In the chart above, count the number of circles in each column and write the total in the spaces at the bottom of the columns. *If you have five or more circles in column 5, you are a Body Type A. If you are not a Body Type A, please continue.*

STEP 3. Look at column 1 and column 2 and determine which of those two columns has the most circles. That column number (1 or 2) is your *primary number*. For example, if the total of column 1 is three and the total of column 2 is five, then your primary number is two. Write your primary number in the box below.

```
┌─────────────────────────────┐
│      PRIMARY NUMBER         │
│                             │
│                             │
└─────────────────────────────┘
```

Note: If you have the same number in columns 1 and 2, your primary number is 1.

STEP 4. Look at column 3 and column 4 and determine which of those two columns has the most circles. That column number is your *secondary number.* Write that number in the box below.

```
┌─────────────────────────────┐
│    SECONDARY NUMBER         │
│                             │
│                             │
└─────────────────────────────┘
```

STEP 5. Use your primary number and your secondary number to identify your body type:

- If your *primary* number is *1* and your *secondary* number is *4,* your *body type* is B.

- If your *primary* number is *1* and your *secondary* number is *3,* your *body type* is C.

- If your *primary* number is *2* and your *secondary* number is *4,* your *body type* is D.

- If your *primary* number is *2* and your *secondary* number is *3,* your *body type* is E.

Write your body type in the box below.

```
┌─────────────────────────────┐
│       MY BODY TYPE          │
│                             │
│                             │
└─────────────────────────────┘
```

Important Note: If you have more than two circles in column 6, you may have a tendency toward low blood sugar, technically known as hypoglycemia. Please read the section on hypoglycemia in appendix B, Customizations for Special Medical Conditions. If you had five or more checks in column 6, you may be very hypoglycemic, and you should consult with your physician before you begin the 6-Day Body Makeover.

In addition, if you checked statement 36, you may have low blood pressure. Please read the information on low blood pressure in appendix B before you start this program. Consult with your physician before beginning the program.

Understanding Your Body Type and Your Metabolism

Now that you've identified your body type, read this section carefully. I list for you the major body composition and metabolic characteristics that correspond to your body type. In parentheses are the technical descriptions of each body type: *endomorph, endo-meso, meso-endo, endo-ecto,* and *ecto-endo.* These terms are derived from a scientific system that classifies the human body into one of three types based on where it deposits fat and how it builds muscle: endomorph (a round, soft shape); mesomorph (muscular and athletic); and ectomorph (a thin shape with smaller bones and joints and little muscle). Although some people are purely endomorph, mesomorph, or ectomorph, most of us are a mixture of body types, with one type being dominant. An endo-meso, for example, is someone who has the characteristics of an endomorph (tends to gain fat easily) but also has quite a bit of lean muscle on his or her body. An ecto-endo is similar to the ectomorph (thin with small bones and joints) but puts on weight as easily as an endomorph.

Regardless of your individual body type, you have the physical potential to develop a beautiful body and an attractive shape through diet and exercise. Knowing your body type is the first step toward attaining those goals.

Each description below is accompanied by an illustration of that particular body type. These are generic sketches of the male and female of that body type and will help you further determine your body type. Don't expect to see an exact match of your body, however. Simply look to see if one of the drawings looks similar to you in terms of where your body gains weight.

Body Type A (Endomorph)

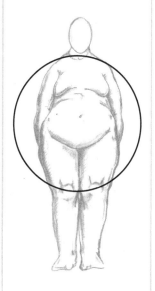

Your body is nearly 100 percent endomorph, with a higher-than-desirable percentage of body fat distributed at and below the waist. Quite probably, you have always had trouble managing your weight and tend to be quite heavy. You put on weight easily, and for the most part you gain it evenly over your entire body. This gives you a softer, rounder physique, with a tendency toward obesity. Other identifying characteristics include:

Body Composition

- Your physique is shaped much like a *circle*—large and round.
- You may be larger around your waist or in your hip and buttocks regions, or even all over your entire body.
- You have more body fat on your frame relative to lean muscle.
- Your muscles are underdeveloped.
- Your body is soft, and your flesh is loose.
- You may have been overweight as a child.

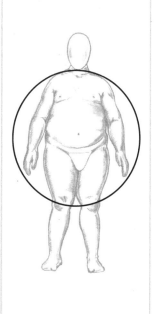

Metabolic Characteristics

- Yours is the slowest metabolism of all five body types.
- You have a tendency to metabolize any food taken into your body as body fat.
- You have a ready disposition toward gaining body fat.
- It is difficult for you to lose body fat.

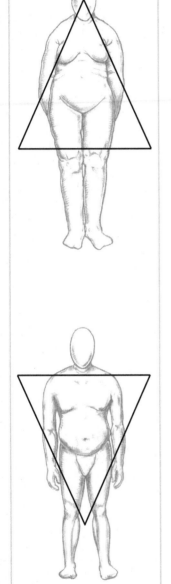

Body Type B (Endo-Meso)

Your dominant body type is endomorph, but with the solid muscular development of a mesomorph. You tend to be thick all over, with loose flesh over the muscle. What's more, you gain weight easily and may be significantly overweight (20 or more pounds). Other identifying characteristics include:

Body Composition

- You may be shaped like a *triangle*, with body fat concentrated in your hips, thighs, and buttocks, particularly if you are a woman.

- You may have narrow shoulders, a small chest, and an average-sized waist.

- You have strong muscle tone beneath your layer of body fat.

Metabolic Characteristics

- You gain fat easily.

- You have trouble losing weight.

- Your metabolism is sluggish.

- You build and maintain muscle easily.

Body Type C (Meso-Endo)

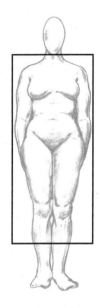

You have a strong, muscular body—the kind you might see on athletes. In other words, mesomorph characteristics are dominant. Yet like an endomorph, you have a difficult time reducing body fat. You tend to gain weight in specific areas rather than evenly all over your body. On parts of your body, oversized muscles are almost as big a problem as having too much body fat. Other identifying characteristics include:

Body Composition

- Your frame is generally thick-bodied. Shape-wise, it may resemble a *rectangle*, roughly the same width at the shoulders, waist, and hips.

- There is a covering of fat over your muscle. (This fat might be intramuscular, like the marbling in red meat.)

- Your body has tight, hard flesh, with fatty tissue covering it.

- You may have broad shoulders.

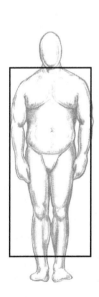

Metabolic Characteristics

- You gain body fat fairly easily.

- Your metabolism is not as sluggish as other body types because of your muscular development.

- You build and maintain muscle tissue very easily.

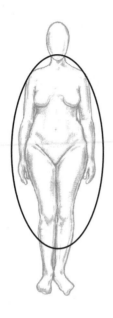

Body Type D (Endo-Ecto)

You may be significantly overweight, inclined to gain weight easily—like an endomorph. Yet you have the slight frame of an ectomorph. You have very little muscle on your body, and your flesh tends to look loose and flabby. Other identifying characteristics include:

Body Composition

- Your shape may resemble an *oval,* with a fuller chest and a less defined waist.

- You may have a skinny body underneath the body fat, with very little muscle tissue.

- You may have a slight frame and are generally small-boned, but over time you've rounded out with a greater percentage of body fat.

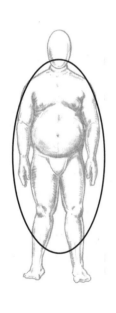

Metabolic Characteristics

- Your metabolism is somewhat more sluggish than other body types.

- You tend to gain weight easily.

- You struggle to build and maintain lean muscle.

Body Type E (Ecto-Endo)

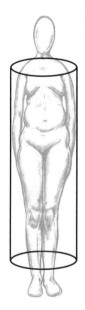

You're essentially a lanky, thin person (like an ectomorph), but you have gained too much weight in places. Your weight problems may be relatively new; at one time, you found it hard to put on weight. You have very little muscle tissue and may actually be skinny or bony on parts of your body, while other parts—your abdomen, waist, or thighs—tend to be overweight with loose, droopy flesh. Other identifying characteristics include:

Body Composition

- Where once your body may have been described as a stick, with a thin, lean look, now you've rounded out, filling out in places, and your physique resembles a *tube*. In other words, there is a skinny, bony frame underneath areas of body fat.

- You have very little muscle tissue.

- You may have skinny arms or legs.

Metabolic Characteristics

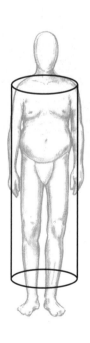

- Your overall metabolic rate is not as slow as other body types, but is still not fast enough to keep you lean.

- It is difficult for you to burn enough calories to keep from gaining weight.

- You have trouble building and maintaining lean muscle.

- At a younger age, you could eat anything you wanted without ever gaining weight.

Can You Change Your Body Type?

Now that you know your body type, you're equipped with the first, and perhaps the most important, piece of the weight-loss puzzle we're putting together here. Hold on to this information, because it will help you put your rapid-weight-loss plan into action.

Because most body types are inherited and genes don't change, we were all born with a basic shape that stays genetically fixed. Even so, you can "remodel" your entire body with a diet and an exercise program customized for your individual body type. Diet and cardiovascular exercise, for example, transform your body by getting rid of unwanted excess fat, by speeding up your metabolism, and by preventing the tendency for your body to gain excess fat as you get older. Exercise that uses weights, bands, or some other form of resistance that challenges your muscles gives you the power to build up or scale down specific areas of your body, thus giving your body more shapely, proportional contours. Thus, you can change your body type to a degree as long as you employ the right mixture of diet and exercise.

In fact, many of my makeover clients started out as one body type, lost excess fat, resculpted their proportions, then took the Blueprinting questionnaire after reaching their goals, only to discover that they were a different body type! Reshaping your body to your exact specifications is a result of losing fat, firming up, and "proportionalizing" muscle. Here's the bottom line, though: Nearly 70 percent of achieving the body you want has to do with diet and nutrition and learning how to use food as a fat-burning tool. That's where we're headed next.

CHAPTER 2

Why It Works: The Metabolic Principles Behind the 6-Day Body Makeover

Y ou're finally going to learn how to lose weight quickly and safely, drop down to a smaller size, and look so much better in your clothes—in six days. The *6-Day Body Makeover* is going to help you succeed. This time will be different.

What exactly will be different? Remember, you're going to follow a plan that is completely customized to you and uses food (lots of it) to burn fat consistently from one day to the next. Because no two people are the same, the eating plan will be different for each individual.

This will not be the kind of crash diet that you may have tried and failed with in the past! It is an easy-to-follow program of healthy, natural, and clean-burning foods. Over the next six days, you will be eating at regular intervals throughout the day, not starving, to lose pounds and inches—and accelerate your metabolism in the process. In this chapter, you'll find out why rapid results are possible when you know how to stop sabotaging yourself with dietary practices that simply do not work.

Peel Off Pounds and Inches: The Seven Metabolic Maximizers for Safe, Accelerated Weight Loss

The reason this program works so effectively is because it is based on sound scientific principles for reprogramming your metabolism to burn more of the food you feed it and store less of it as body fat. When you eat a meal, your body either dismantles it and burns it for fuel or stores it away greedily as fat (or as glycogen, a storage form of carbohydrate, in your muscles) for later use as an energy source. Both modes—storing and burning—go on simultaneously, although one mode usually prevails, depending upon how efficient your metabolism is. Suffice to say, if yours is a pokey metabolism, your body is in mostly a storage mode and you gain weight; if yours is a fast metabolism, it is in mostly a burning mode and you lose weight. Naturally, you want to set your metabolic tempo on "burn"—to manipulate your metabolism so that you burn up whatever you feed your body. When you do that—change your metabolism from pokey to supercharged—accelerated weight loss is practically automatic.

What follows is a look at the major metabolic principles that allow you to set the controls on burn. Once you understand these principles and apply them, you'll be able to start reprogramming your metabolism to drop a size in six days. What's more, if you incorporate these principles into an ongoing weight-management program, you'll ultimately be able to keep your weight at whatever level you want for the rest of your life.

> *"The last 10 pounds have been a battle for me all of my life! Thanks to the 6-Day Body Makeover, I lost 10 pounds, 2 inches from my hips, and 4 inches off my waist! Most importantly, I did not have to resort to drastic measures to achieve these results. I never thought that I could eat so much and yet be able to still lose weight. Finally, I have the body I have always wanted!"*
>
> *—Parissa*

One: Emphasize Slow Carbohydrates Over Fast Carbohydrates

The cereal you had for breakfast, the bread you ate in your sandwich at lunch, the apple you snacked on—these are all examples of carbohydrates, or "carbs." However you choose to think of them, carbohydrates are to your body what gas is to your car—the fuel that gets you going. During digestion, carbs break down to sugar in your body to fuel your muscles and your brain. Assisted by the metabolic hormone insulin, this sugar (glucose) is then escorted into cells to be used by various tissues in your body. Among other tasks, insulin is responsible for regulating glucose levels in your body.

Once it's inside a cell, glucose can be quickly metabolized to supply energy. Or it can be converted to either liver or muscle glycogen and stored for later use. When you exercise or use your muscles in any way, your body mobilizes glycogen initially for energy. If you overindulge in carbohydrates—that is, eat more than your body can burn up or store as glycogen—the excess gets stored as body fat.

In addition to supplying necessary fuel for your body, carbs are the only source of a nutrient called fiber. Fiber is the nondigestible remnant of carbohydrates, and it passes through your digestive system relatively intact. Fiber is what keeps you "regular." But it also aids in weight control—in two major ways: Fiber provides satisfying bulk that makes you feel naturally full, and it pushes food through your system faster so that less calories and fat are absorbed. Whole grains, beans and legumes, fruits, and vegetables are the best sources of health-building fiber.

Although there are several ways carbohydrates are classified, I make a distinction between "fast carbs" and "slow carbs," the basic difference having to do with how quickly they are broken down and converted into sugar in the body.

Fast carbs (often termed simple carbohydrates) are transformed to sugar very quickly by your body. This category includes sweet foods such as table sugar, candy, honey, molasses, sugary desserts, cakes, cookies, fruit juice, sugared sodas, certain types of sweet fruits, and all processed carbs (bread, bread products, pasta, sugared cereals, and so forth).

Slow carbs (also termed complex carbohydrates) are converted to sugar much more slowly by your body. Examples of slow carbs include potatoes, sweet potatoes, yams, whole-grain cereals, vegetables, and low-sugar fruits.

While following the *6-Day Body Makeover*, you must swear off fast carbohydrates, particularly all forms of processed carbs (unless you are very hypoglycemic—see appendix B for information). These foods overstimulate the release of insulin in your body. At normal levels, insulin is a vital hormone, with many important functions in the body. But when repeatedly elevated by an excess of fast carbs, insulin activates fat cell enzymes that herd fat from your bloodstream into fat cells for storage and trigger your body to create even more fat cells. Insulin at high levels thus becomes a fat-forming hormone, creating a chemical reaction that can slow your metabolism so dramatically that it will actually prevent your body from burning stored fat. Even one serving of a fast carb can spike your insulin to the point that your body stops burning fat. Simply put, fast carbs are rapid inducers of insulin. Eliminating them helps accelerate weight loss.

Fast carbs such as simple sugars do have their uses, however. If you are experiencing hypoglycemic symptoms (low blood sugar), a simple sugar can restore proper blood sugar levels quickly. I've often advised clients on my makeover programs to immediately eat something sweet, such as raisins or fruit juice, in order to stabilize themselves when they experience the shakiness and weakness associated with low blood sugar. But for most weight-loss purposes, slow carbs are a far better choice.

The carbohydrate emphasis on my *6-Day Body Makeover* is thus on mostly slow carbohydrates. Among these, the most beneficial for accelerated weight loss are yams, sweet potatoes, beans, quinoa, and certain types of rice (particularly wild rice, brown rice, and long-grain rice). The reason is that these carbs turn to sugar much more slowly than fast carbs, meaning that there is less of an insulin spike with its corresponding metabolic drop. Although potatoes are technically a fast carb, they're also included— for several reasons. First, potatoes are a natural source of potassium, which helps regulate water balance in the body. Second, they're an effective source of energy for exercise. And third, potatoes are filling and thus hunger satisfying.

To further slow carbohydrates' conversion to sugar, you must combine it with another type of food—protein. Combining carbs with protein slows your digestion for a steady, even release of energy. So it is very important to combine your foods properly. The meal plans in chapter 4 do this for you, automatically.

As you will shortly learn, people differ with regard to the types and amounts of carbs they can tolerate. This is one of the primary differences among the eating plans in the *6-Day Body Makeover*.

No matter what your metabolism, if you eat too many carbohydrates in one meal, you run the risk of elevating your insulin levels and shutting down your metabolism.

Does this mean the *6-Day Body Makeover* eating plans are low carb? Absolutely not! Let me reiterate: Low-carb diets in which you virtually eliminate carbs and jack up your protein consumption can jeopardize your ability to lose weight and achieve a sculpted, sexy body. If carbs are in short supply, your body is forced to draw on its lean muscle tissue (protein) for energy, a potentially dangerous situation. When your body must break down its own protein for fuel, this vital nutrient is not available for building and replacing body tissues such as muscle. In fact, you will lose body-firming muscle rather than unsightly body fat on low-carb diets! Muscle is metabolically active, too, so losing it means your metabolism will run in very low gear. It is important to add that body fat burns more efficiently and completely in the presence of carbohydrates. You need carbs!

It is clear that low-carb diets—the current hot diet fad—go against the grain of proper metabolic functioning for weight loss. On the *6-Day Body Makeover,* you'll be following a more nutrient-balanced plan—not shortchanging yourself on carbs. Your body will burn more of your stored fat (which is exactly what you want to burn) than any other bodily component. Eating the right carbs in the right amounts for your metabolism is one of the critical factors that makes this happen.

Two: Include Lean High-Quality Protein at Most Meals

For shedding pounds and trimming inches, it is of paramount importance that you eat an adequate amount of high-quality protein each day. Protein is the only nutrient directly responsible for building lean, shapely muscle—so you want to choose the very best sources. The best and most efficient way to get this type of protein is from lean animal sources—chicken, fish, meat, and egg whites. It is more of a challenge to obtain enough protein from plant sources, such as soy, legumes, or nuts. These foods are lower in certain amino acids, the building blocks of protein that are used to form new tissues and replace worn-out ones, and your body therefore cannot take full advantage of these foods as protein sources to support continued growth and repair.

Not only does protein play a vital role in creating every beautiful piece of firm, curvaceous muscle, but it can also speed up the fat-burning process. Protein happens to have the highest thermic effect of any food because it requires more energy to digest and absorb than either carbohydrate or fat, and this stimulates your metabolism. In fact, eating protein at meals can speed up your metabolic rate considerably—by as much as 30 percent. Translated, this means that out of 100 calories of a protein food like chicken breast, the net amount of calories left over after processing it is 70.

On many fad diets, you're advised to "eat all you want" of protein because protein is less likely to be converted to fat than any other nutrient. While it is true that protein is not well stored, it is false that you can eat it in unlimited amounts. Too much of any food

IF YOU'RE A VEGETARIAN

As a vegetarian, you can still follow the *6-Day Body Makeover*. While it is harder to get protein from nonanimal sources, it is not impossible. The three primary vegetarian protein choices that I recommend are egg whites, tofu, and protein drinks. To use them on your plan, substitute 4 egg whites or 4 ounces of tofu for 4 ounces of animal protein; 3 egg whites or 3 ounces of tofu for 3 ounces of animal protein; or 2 egg whites or 2 ounces of tofu for animal protein, depending on the amount your eating plan calls for. The one caution about tofu is that it contains estrogen, a hormone that can slow down your weight loss.

If you want to use powdered protein, I recommend a combination of 1 scoop whey protein isolate and 1 scoop soy protein isolate. This represents one 4-ounce serving of protein in your eating plan. Add it to a bowl of oatmeal or prepare it in water. You also have the option of using textured vegetable protein (TVP) or other meat substitutes, available in most health food stores and supermarkets. *Warning:* Pay attention to the amount of sodium and sugar in these products and try to find the one that has the least amount of these additives. TVP can substitute ounce for ounce for the animal protein on your eating plan.

type can be stored as body fat, including protein. Proteins are assimilated by the body in small amounts. You cannot scarf down a 16-ounce slice of prime rib for dinner a few nights a week and expect to lose weight. Four ounces of protein per meal is about the limit. Eat more than that, and you run the risk of storing the excess as body fat.

Here's something else about protein you won't learn on other "diets": *Different proteins have different rates of utilization.* Your body will metabolize, or burn up, white fish such as sole or flounder more quickly than a heavy red meat. Lean poultry metabolizes rapidly, too, and egg whites metabolize even faster than fish or poultry. Incorporating proteins that metabolize quickly is one of the prime components of the eating plans on the *6-Day Body Makeover*.

At this point, you're probably wondering: *How much protein do I really need?* The amount of protein each person requires is basically determined by your sex and by your body type. Your body type speaks volumes about your metabolism, whether it is slow, slower, or somewhere in between. Thus, your protein allowances at each meal are designed to match your metabolism so that you have adequate protein to maintain muscle or increase it, plus burn fat faster. As you will see in the next chapter, I've designed each meal plan to fulfill your personal protein requirements. All the calculations are done for you; all you have to do is carefully weigh your allotted protein portions. Rest assured that your customized meal plan is designed with the optimum type and quantity of protein for your individual metabolism.

Three: The Fat You Eat Is the Fat You Wear

You know what really irks me? When people who sincerely want to lose weight go on one of these high-fat diets, and I have to tell them they've been conned! These diets are thoroughly unsound and out of sync with what you need to keep your metabolism at peak function. Before you sabotage yourself with one of these high-fat diets, let me talk straight with you: Fats are fattening! If you really want to lose weight—and ultimately keep it off—you must keep your dietary fats to a bare minimum.

Here's the deal: Fats are stored in your body far more readily than either carbohydrates or protein. The reason is that very little energy is expended to assimilate dietary fat compared with these other nutrients. As noted above, your body works very hard to

> *"I've gone from a size 12 to a size 2 or 4, using Michael's makeover techniques, including the 6-Day Body Makeover. I've lost 6 inches in my waist, 8 inches in my hips, and 5 inches in each thigh. I've probably been on every diet in the world . . . and eventually I gained all the weight back. With Michael's programs . . . the weight seemed to melt off and it's four years later and it's still off."*
>
> *—Sharon*

break down protein—and almost as hard to break down carbs—but it doesn't work hard to break down fat. It takes a long time for your body to metabolize fat, or turn it into fuel, so there is a greater chance of it being stored—as fat. In fact, your body recognizes dietary fat as fat and prefers to hang on to it rather than break it down for energy—storing it around your belly, on your hips or thighs, or wherever it is that your particular body type tends to deposit fat. This affinity your body has for storing dietary fat has a detrimental effect on your metabolism, too. An excess of fat in your diet can actually slow down your metabolism, making it difficult to lose weight and easier for you to pack on unwanted pounds.

Minimizing the fat in your diet will help you shed pounds not just in the short term but over the long haul as well. Very powerful proof from the National Weight Control Registry, an ongoing research study of more than 4,000 individuals who have lost significant amounts of weight and kept it off for long periods of time, indicates that controlling dietary fat intake is a key strategy for long-term management of body weight. The message in this very important study: Control your fat intake and you'll keep your weight in check, quite possibly for a lifetime. The results I've witnessed in my own makeover clients—those who have kept their weight off for years—underscores the value of monitoring dietary fat and keeping it to a minimum in your diet.

Certainly, fat is a fuel source, like carbohydrates, but it has to be first stored as additional fat before it is burned. The trick to burning as much body fat as possible is an exercise technique called long slow distance exercise, which you'll learn about in chapter 5. It is the most efficient way to burn stored fat as fuel.

I'm sure you've heard that fats are often described as being "bad fats" or "good fats"—terms that basically refer to saturated fats and unsaturated fats. Generally solid at room temperature, saturated fats include butter, cream cheese, lard, tropical oils, the marbled fat in beef, and hydrogenated fats found in margarine, shortening, and peanut butter. Saturated fats are responsible for elevating levels of artery-clogging cholesterol in the bloodstream.

Unsaturated fats are generally liquid at room temperature and are derived from plant sources. Certain types of unsaturated fats are considered healthier than saturated fats. However, as far as weight loss is concerned, fat is still fat. The body has an affinity for fat, regardless of its saturation, and will store fat before it stores carbohydrates or protein. In addition, 1 gram of fat has 9 calories—more than twice the caloric content of an equivalent amount of carbohydrate or protein. The belief that fat goes from the mouth to the stomach to the hips, while not physiologically true, is not without some basis in fact.

We do need some fat in our diets for the healthy functioning of our bodies, for the absorption of certain vitamins, for normal blood clotting, and for protecting the membranes that surround our cells—but not to the degree that most Americans consume fat. There is no need to add it to your food! You can obtain all the fat you need from eating very lean meats and fish—foods that naturally contain fat. You will not deprive yourself of anything by cutting way back on fat.

The *6-Day Body Makeover* is designed to be low in fat in order to coax your body into a fat-burning mode. During this program, you're going to eliminate as much fat as possible. By doing so, you'll be able to achieve the quick results you're looking for. Any kind of added oils or fat will dramatically affect your progress. This is only a six-day program—so you have to be very vigilant about this. Remember: Fat can cause weight gain. For weight loss and general good health, you must limit the amount of fat you consume.

"Yesterday I bought a pair of size 14 pants from a women's specialty store. My friend who works there said, 'You won't be able to shop here much longer because a size 14 is the smallest we carry.' That was music to my ears." —*Melba*

Four: Deemphasize Sodium for Accelerated Weight Loss

Here is something else that may surprise you: One of the unrecognized keys to fast yet safe weight loss is to control the amount of sodium you consume. You know sodium best as table salt, but salt and sodium are hidden in all kinds of products, including packaged foods, fast foods, sodas, frozen and canned foods, condiments, and other food products. No matter where it hides out, excess sodium in your diet will dramatically slow down your metabolism.

How is this possible? The answer is water retention. When you eat more salt than you need, some of the extra sodium is deposited just beneath your skin. There it attracts water, which is retained in your cells. This watery logjam not only adds pounds, but also distorts the shape of your body and keeps you from getting even your "fat" clothes to fit. You look and feel puffy, miserable, and uncomfortable because it feels like you've gained 10 pounds or more.

As your body metabolizes, or burns, fat, the by-product is water. In order to make the fat-burning process as efficient as possible, your body requires a steady flow of fluid in and out of your body. If water gets dammed up in your cells, this flow is obstructed, thus making you bloated. Think of it this way: Slowing the flow out is like putting a potato in the tailpipe of your car; it dramatically reduces the efficiency of the engine. Similarly, sodium-induced water retention has the potential to dramatically slow or stop your body's engine—your metabolism.

While this may sound disheartening, there is one simple way to get rid of the cause of bloating and impaired metabolism: Put down the saltshaker and avoid foods containing a lot of sodium! For the six days of this program, you must totally eliminate salt from your diet, unless you have low blood pressure, which we will discuss later. This means trading in processed foods for fresh, homemade foods, since almost all precooked meats, including lunch meats and packaged foods, are loaded with sodium. Even rotisserie-cooked chicken is generally loaded with both sodium and fat. Go to the health food or grocery store and buy only the freshest foods possible. Stay away from prepackaged foods during this program as well.

True, we need some sodium in our diets, but most people eat too much. In fact, we need only about a tenth of a teaspoon a day! Fortunately, salt is present naturally in just about every type of food. So if you eat a normal amount of food, you'll almost certainly get all the salt you need. But what if you have a "salt tooth"? Don't worry: Once you start cutting down on salt, you'll lose your taste for it.

Many foods are higher in sodium than others. Of course, common table salt is the highest. I've listed other high-sodium foods for you in the chart below (the higher the food is on the list, the higher its sodium content). These foods are not included on my makeover programs.

BAKED PRODUCTS

Baking powder

BEVERAGES

Carbonated beverages (with the exception of sodium-free soft drinks)
Club soda

Carbonated beverages, sugar-free, with sodium saccharin
Unsweetened soft drink mix, powder

DAIRY AND EGG PRODUCTS

Egg yolk, raw, frozen, salted
Cheeses

FATS AND OILS

Italian salad dressing, fat-free
Margarine-like spread, fat-free
Blue cheese salad dressing, reduced fat
Italian salad dressing, reduced fat
Sweet-and-sour salad dressing
Margarine spread, fat-free, tub

Mayonnaise dressing, fat-free
Caesar salad dressing, low calorie
Mayonnaise-like spread, fat-free or low calorie
Peanut butter
Salted butter

FOODS HIGHEST IN SODIUM

FAST FOODS

Green beans (side order)
Vegetable beef soup
Minestrone

Chicken noodle soup
Ham salad

FISH AND SHELLFISH

Clams, canned
Dried fish
Anchovies, canned in oil

Smoked salmon (lox)
Alaska king crab
Fish, smoked

LEGUMES AND LEGUME PRODUCTS

Soy sauce
Soy sauce, low sodium
Tofu, salted

Miso
Beans, canned

SAUSAGES AND LUNCH MEATS

Beef, cured and dried
Ham, smoked, fat-free
Chicken breast, oven roasted,
   fat-free
Turkey breast, smoked, fat-free
Fat-free hot dogs

Ham luncheon meat, including
   fat-free
Bologna, fat-free
Ham, extra lean
Corned beef

SPICES AND HERBS

Capers, canned
Mustard, prepared, yellow
Garlic salt

Onion salt
Seasonings such as lemon pepper

SOUPS, SAUCES, AND GRAVIES

Fish sauce

Consommé, dry or prepared with water, or ready-to-serve

Beef broth or bouillon, dry or prepared with water, or ready-to-serve

Oyster sauce

Virtually all soups, canned, dehydrated, or ready-to-serve

Salsa, bottled

Worcestershire sauce

Gravy, canned

Gravy, instant, dry

SWEETS

Puddings, fat-free and sugar-free

Cakes

VEGETABLES AND VEGETABLE PRODUCTS

Pickles, cucumber, sour or dill

Peppers, jalapeños, canned

Peppers, hot chile, red or green, canned

Grape leaves, canned

Sauerkraut, canned

Canned vegetables

Tomato juice, canned

Vegetable juice cocktail, canned

Sauerkraut, canned, low sodium

Pickle relish

Catsup

There is no set amount of sodium to be consumed in a day. You should only be ingesting sodium from the natural food sources listed in your eating plan, unless your doctor has instructed you to do otherwise. Because the level of naturally occurring sodium varies by what foods you choose to eat, the amount of sodium that you get daily will vary.

For seasoning your foods without salt, Mrs. Dash, McCormick Salt Free Seasoning, and Spice Hunter are all good choices. So is salsa, as long as it's homemade (see page 203 for a recipe). Most health food stores carry salt-free seasoning blends that are perfect for all types of foods. Always read the label to make sure they do not contain salt or sugar. In many lemon-pepper seasonings, for example, the first ingredient on the label is salt, so always check the ingredients list. Also, don't underestimate the flavor of pepper. Pepper naturally adds more flavor to food than salt does—and without masking the taste of the food. Freshly ground pepper is the best choice because it tastes so much better than the kind you buy in the shaker.

Food can be flavorful without salt as long as you spice it up with spices and herbs, too. There's another advantage to this besides flavor: Spicy foods accelerate your metabolic rate. When people eat hot peppers, chili, or cayenne pepper, they often sweat. That's a sign of a revved-up metabolic rate. The faster your metabolic rate, the more heat your body produces, and whatever heats up your body helps trim you down. The message here is: Learn to use spices such as chili powder, red pepper, curry, and others in your cooking, particularly in place of salt. Salt actually makes you eat more than you should and has a detrimental effect on metabolism. So get rid of the saltshaker and turn to the spice rack instead (again, unless you have low blood pressure—90/60 or lower).

One of the main reasons people put so much salt on their food is because food sometimes tastes so bland. The solution is to make your food taste better naturally, so you won't miss the salt. For anyone trying to eat healthy, citrus fruits such as lemons and limes are a godsend. They mix well with almost any ingredients, taste delicious, and are completely fat-free. And they're versatile, working equally well on meats, vegetables, and salads. You can even add a squirt of lemon juice to plain water for a delicious, refreshing flavor. If keeping fresh lemons or limes on hand is inconvenient, many supermarkets sell presqueezed natural lemon and lime juice. Look for a small plastic bottle in the shape of a lemon or lime.

Recommended herbs and spices, used individually or in combination, are listed below:

Basil	*Dill*	*Oregano*
Cayenne	*Fresh garlic*	*Paprika*
Chervil	*Garlic powder*	*Parsley*
Chili powder	*Ginger*	*Pepper*
Cilantro	*Lemon juice*	*Rosemary*
Coriander	*Marjoram*	*Sage*
Cumin	*Mint*	*Tarragon*
Curry	*Onion powder*	*Thyme*

Without a doubt, eliminating added sodium is one of the simplest ways to boost weight loss. You'll be delighted to see your body lose pounds and inches steadily, as you make this simple change.

Five: Go with Greens and Other Diuretic Vegetables for Extra Slimming Benefits

Another of my trade secrets for accelerated weight loss: greens. Green vegetables are technically another form of carbohydrates, although they supply very little food energy in the way of calories. They do offer other weight-control benefits, however. One of their advantages is that greens are naturally diuretic. They increase the flow of fluid from the body—as I discussed above—and therefore help prevent the metabolic down-shift that can lead to bloating. Green vegetables are endowed with the mineral potassium, which actually helps prevent fluid retention. This action helps to reduce blood pressure, as well as to remove impurities from your system. Greens include spinach, lettuce (all varieties), mustard greens, parsley, collard greens, beet greens, turnip greens, kale, dandelion greens, arugula, and watercress.

In addition to these foods, some of the best diuretic vegetables include asparagus and cucumbers. If you've snubbed asparagus in the past, you may want to rethink your position. Asparagus is an excellent natural diuretic, so if you tend to bloat, select this vegetable at several meals throughout the next six days. It is also brimming with folic acid, a B vitamin involved in preventing heart disease.

Among fruits and vegetables, cucumbers probably contain the most water—nearly 96 percent and virtually no calories (14 per cup). Added to salads, they fill you up and make great snacks.

Greens, in general, also supply generous doses of vitamins, minerals, antioxidants, phytochemicals, and fiber—all known to promote good health. For the six days of your makeover, you'll eat greens in measured portions. But afterward, as my clients do on my *6-Week Body Makeover*, you can generally eat all the greens you want.

I realize that many people detest green vegetables. My goal is not to force-feed you greens and make you hate them, but to help you enjoy them more. If you don't like kale, then don't eat it. You can have spinach or romaine lettuce or something else to get the same benefits. Any eating plan that denies our basic need for pleasure will eventually fail—so take what you like and fit it into your plan. That's important because ultimately you'll want to go from this six-day plan to a plan for the rest of your life.

Six: Eat Multiple Meals Spaced at Regular Intervals Throughout the Day

When and how often you eat are just as important as what you eat. On the *6-Day Body Makeover*, you eat more than you've ever eaten on any other diet, because the key to this program is just that: eating. The first thing you'll notice when you start this makeover is that there are six meals—breakfast, midmorning snack, lunch, midafternoon snack, dinner, and a PM or evening snack. That's six meals a day, every day. Right away, you can see how different this is from a lot of the diets you may have tried in the past. On this program, you eat, and you eat a lot. And *you must eat for this program to work*.

Not only do you eat multiple meals, but you must also space your meals two to three hours apart. This eating schedule activates the burning off of stored fat in your body. Eating frequently throughout the day boosts your metabolism because the digestive process burns calories as heat is given off. Thus, the more often you eat, the more your metabolism stays cranked up.

When you eat more often, your body learns that it is always going to get food when it needs it. So it stops worrying that it may starve. It stops storing the calories you eat and makes it all available to burn as energy. And that is the goal of this makeover—to speed up your metabolism to the point that it burns more calories than you consume. That's when you lose weight. Eating all the food allotted to you is very important to your success.

With multiple meals, your body receives a constant stream of energy-giving nutrients. Eating more frequently helps your body better utilize vitamins, minerals, and other nutrients. The net effect is that you'll feel energized as you go through the day—more pep and less fatigue. Multiple meals also tame your cravings. You're less likely to get hungry or be tempted to veer from the plan.

As a preview of coming attractions, let me walk you through your meal schedule on the *6-Day Body Makeover*.

Your first meal of the day is breakfast, which usually consists of a protein and some-

IN WAYS YOU CAN LOVE

It's no secret that vegetables are the healthiest foods around, packed with vitamins, minerals, antioxidants, phytochemicals, and fiber—and that we need to up our intake for lifelong health and weight control. But the problem is: Far too many people just hate vegetables and refuse even to try to choke them down.

If you're a vegetable hater, listen up! There are ways to make nature's healthiest foods taste delicious. One method is to spice them right. Here's the rundown on which spices work best with certain vegetables and greens:

Broccoli or brussels sprouts: Caraway seeds

Green beans: Tarragon or dill weed

Spinach: Nutmeg

Squash: Allspice or curry

Tomatoes: Basil, oregano, red pepper, or rosemary

Green, red, or yellow peppers: Thyme

Two other suggestions include dipping raw vegetables in homemade salsa (the recipe is on page 203), or trying the "baby versions" of certain vegetables such as artichokes, turnips, or squash (they tend to be more flavorful and less bitter).

times a fresh fruit, depending on your individualized menu. If you have developed the habit of not eating breakfast, that spells trouble, since people who skip breakfast tend to have problems keeping their weight under control. Breakfast is important because it normalizes blood sugar levels during the morning, and gives you the energy and focus you need to start the day. If you skip breakfast, you begin your day in a starvation mode, which is a fat-storing mode!

Now is the time to start eating breakfast on a regular basis. Remember, on this program, you have to eat. You use food to lose weight. So if the idea of eating breakfast is foreign to you, think of it this way: The minute you eat your first meal, that's the minute your metabolism starts speeding up. And your body starts to burn fat.

Two to three hours after breakfast, you'll eat your next meal of the day: your mid-morning snack, a filling meal of protein and greens, or a carbohydrate, depending on your custom eating plan. You may think that eating six meals a day is a huge amount of food, even too much, but because these foods are specifically chosen and proportioned for your body type, your body will process them quickly as fuel, and you'll find yourself hungry again when it's time for your next meal. Listen to your body. When you start to feel hungry, then eat.

Two to three hours after your snack, it's lunchtime. In the middle of the day, you'll need to have a full meal, so along with protein and a vegetable you'll have some sort of carbohydrate, either rice, or a potato or yam, or beans. Keep in mind that your food choices for lunch and other meals are tailored to your unique metabolism.

Then, in the middle of the afternoon, it's time to eat again. This meal consists of a protein and greens, or protein, a fresh fruit, or a carbohydrate.

Your dinner has basically the same components as your lunch: a protein, vegetables, and a carbohydrate.

Your last meal of the day is your PM snack, which may include a fruit, a protein, a vegetable, or some combination of these foods, depending on your customized eating plan. This is the only meal of the day that is optional. As the day comes to a close, your level of activity will probably drop, and you're not going to be able to metabolize much food as your body slows down for the night. But some people get very hungry for a snack in the evening, and this is for them.

Frequent eating, with special combinations of food and at specific times of the day, minimizes your cravings so that you'll feel them less powerfully, or not at all. Once you start eating five to six times a day, you will quickly discover that your cravings and urges to eat fattening foods will lose their grip over you. One reason you might have failed on previous diets is that the diet let you get too hungry, making it easy to cave in to temptation. That won't happen on the *6-Day Body Makeover*, simply because you are eating every two to three hours. In fact, every time you feel hungry, you will eat, but you'll be eating foods that are right for your body chemistry—not the junk food that made you overweight in the past.

Seven: Water Your Body

We have talked generally about what to eat. Now let's talk about what to drink. For the next six days, your primary beverage should be water—in the amount of 12 full glasses a day, or approximately 100 ounces, while following the *6-Day Body Makeover* plan. *This is a simple secret that will accelerate your fat loss.*

I know what you're probably saying: "Michael, that's a lot of water! I can't drink that much!" But hear me out on this: Drinking more water can actually help reduce body fat. Here is the reason why: Your kidneys rely on water to do their job of filtering waste products and impurities from your body. With a water shortage, the kidneys cannot function properly, so they dump their workload on the liver. Among the liver's many functions is metabolizing stored fat into usable fuel for your body. But if your liver has to take on an extra assignment from the kidneys, its ability to burn fat is severely compromised. If less fat is metabolized, more of it remains stored, and weight loss stops. You must drink enough water to help your body metabolize stored fat.

Drinking enough water each day also helps prevent fluid retention. When your body gets less water than it requires, it perceives this shortage as a threat to survival and will start hoarding water. This survival response shows up in swollen feet, hands, and legs, and an overall distorted body shape and extra poundage in the form of retained water. And as I explained earlier, fluid retention interferes with metabolism.

In addition, it is essential that you drink water before, during, and after exercise. Water assists in muscle stimulation by helping your muscles contract. Replenishing water lost through working out helps guard against dehydration and fluid retention.

As for what type of water to drink, I always recommend distilled water because it is sodium-free, although other bottled waters are acceptable, too.

Toward a Smaller Size

Your motivation to stick with the *6-Day Body Makeover* and go on to make other positive dietary changes will come from your own body and mind. Unlike most diets that offer an insufficient supply of critical nutrients, this plan supplies vitamins, minerals, antioxidants, and phytochemicals for nutritional support. Thus, you'll begin to feel better, physically and mentally, and more energetic after just a day or two. When you begin to see your progress on the bathroom scale, this will give you the inspiration to keep going, especially since your body is now being programmed to shed fat and get healthier.

Important: This is an aggressive weight-loss plan designed to take weight off very quickly. Before beginning this, or any other weight-loss program, it is critical to consult your physician or health care provider, particularly if you are taking any medication or have any special medical conditions. If you suffer from hypoglycemia, high or low blood pressure, or food allergies, make sure you also read appendix B, Customizations for Special Medical Conditions, before you start. This will help you adjust your plan to your special body chemistry so that you may achieve maximum results.

Because you now have some powerful knowledge about foods that can help you burn fat and trim down, and understand how the body responds to certain types of food, you are now ready to take this insight to the next level: learning how to eat for your body type and individual metabolism so that you can eat more and lose unwanted weight and inches in just six days.

CHAPTER 3

The 6-Day Body Makeover *Basics*

hat I'd like to talk to you about right now are some general, straightforward rules of how to approach your individual eating plan—and how to be successful while following it. The actual eating plans and menus will follow in the next chapter.

The *6-Day Body Makeover* is simple and doable—after all, anyone can stick to something for six days—and it *is* easy, as long as you follow your eating plan and don't play fast and loose with the rules. If you follow the instructions here and throughout the rest of the book, you *will* succeed, and you'll be amazed at the changes that can take place in your body in just six days.

Basic *6-Day Body Makeover* Rules

1. Follow the eating plan that matches your body type. There are five different eating plans; each one corresponds to a specific body type. For example, if you are a Body Type A, you should follow the Body Type A Makeover Eating Plan. Make sure you follow the plan designated for your body type. Your individual plan is designed expressly for you—to speed up your metabolism and get your body in gear for burning fat very quickly.

For each of the five body types, you'll find a sample eating plan "template" that shows you exactly what types of foods you can eat for each day of the week. You can create your own meal plan by simply interchanging any of your permissible foods in the proper proportions and in the proper meals. This template is a useful tool if you prefer to design your own menus, picking and choosing foods from the food lists. On the other hand, if you prefer to follow an exact plan, then you'll be comfortable using the day-by-day eating plan for your body type. This tells you precisely what to eat at every meal for the entire six days of the program and takes the guesswork out of meal planning. Or you may want to use a combination of these two approaches: creating some of your own daily meals, as well as using the predesigned menus from the day-by-day plan on other days. Whatever approach you use, make sure you follow the plan for your body type!

For variety, you have the option of spicing up your menus using the makeover recipes, which are found in appendix A and used in the eating plans. You'll probably want to read through the recipes, beginning on page 183, for inspiration and ideas.

2. Never skip a meal. You'll be eating five to six times a day, with your meals spaced two to three hours apart. Eating all the food required on the *6-Day Body Makeover* is very important to your success. If you're used to conventional diets, you may think cutting calories works effectively—that if you cut back and eat less, you will lose even faster—but this is not how this plan works. The fact of the matter is: If you skip meals or reduce your portion sizes, the makeover will *not* work.

The first meal on all five menu plans is breakfast. I've mentioned this before, but it's worth repeating: If you normally don't eat breakfast, now is the time to start. Remember, on this program, you must eat. You use food to lose weight. The minute you eat your first meal is the minute your metabolism starts speeding up.

Your sixth and last meal of the day is an optional evening snack. In the evening, your body is naturally slowing down, and you won't be able to metabolize food as quickly. If you're not hungry, you may skip this meal. But other than that, it's very important to eat all your meals. Food is the fuel that keeps your metabolism churning, and the more consistently it works, the faster you lose weight. One of the reasons that people find it difficult to get rid of excess weight is that they don't eat enough. The body reacts as though you were starving, slowing down its metabolism and holding on to the fat, just like a hibernating bear. When you eat consistently, the body processes the food for energy, knowing that in a very short time it will get another portion of food. This is what increases your body metabolism and gets the body to burn the stored fat.

In my years of working with people, I sometimes hear the complaint, "I'm not hungry at mealtimes." This usually happens if you aren't eating your meals on a regular schedule. When you consistently eat every two to three hours, your metabolism will accelerate, and you will start to get hungrier much more often. This is a sign that the program is working. Make a commitment to adhering to your eating plan for the next six days, and this problem should disappear.

Sometimes the unexpected comes up, however, and you can't help but miss a meal. If that happens, just eat your next meal as soon as you can, and get back into the routine of eating. Your metabolism will start back up again in no time.

3. Stick to permissible foods. Each customized menu plan carries with it a list of permissible foods: proteins, carbohydrates, vegetables, greens, and fruits. If a food is not on your list, don't eat it!

You should notice immediately that milk and milk products are not included on the *6-Day Body Makeover*. All of these foods happen to be very high in simple sugars, and some are high in fat. Thus, they have the ability to slow down your metabolism and dramatically reduce weight loss. The purpose of cow's milk is to fatten up baby cows, and it has essentially the same effect on your body: Milk and high-fat dairy foods can actually slow your metabolism. For these reasons alone, you should avoid these foods while following the *6-Day Body Makeover*. The only time I incorporate dairy foods into someone's makeover program is if the client is a child or teen. Dairy foods are among the primary foods children and teenagers need for growth.

Sugar and sugar-laced foods are not included, either. Sugar slows down your metabolism, too, so you must avoid it. If you have a sweet tooth, expect your craving for sweets to subside after just a few days on the *6-Day Body Makeover*. That is because you are fueling your body with pure, natural foods and cleansing it of additives such as added sugar (the number one additive in processed foods today). If you really crave something sweet, make sure you eat your optional PM evening snack, which in most cases allows fresh fruit. If you still find yourself craving sweets, satisfy that craving with a diet soda. However, be aware that most diet sodas are high in sodium, so you run the risk of slowing your weight loss due to water retention. Certain diet sodas have no sodium; Diet Rite is one such brand. Another suggestion is to try some of the dessert recipes I've included for you in appendix A.

You may also use sweeteners, as long as they don't contain any sodium. That means no saccharin. Splenda and Equal are the preferred sweeteners to use because they are least offensive to your body. Another good natural sweetener is the herb stevia. Look for it in your health food store. For an extra hint of sweetness, you may also use extracts such as vanilla or almond extract, or cinnamon.

4. Always select lean proteins. The protein you eat is always noted as being lean. This is very important. If your plan calls for chicken breast, make sure you get only breast meat and only the skinless type. The same goes for turkey. Skin contains a large portion of fat. Also, be sure to use white meat poultry and only the leanest part. Trim excess fat from all meat. Make sure there are no other additives to the chicken or turkey breast—no chicken broth, nothing. Often when you buy big packages of frozen breast meat, whether it's chicken or turkey, it's injected with high-sodium chicken broth or turkey broth to enhance the meat's flavor. You'll want to avoid these products.

5. Be mindful of the portion sizes on your eating plan. For the *6-Day Body Makeover* to work, you must pay strict attention to your portions—the amount of protein, carbohydrates, vegetables, greens, and fruits you eat at each meal. This is important, since certain nutrients are not assimilated or converted into fuel when eaten in excess amounts, wreaking havoc on your metabolism.

Women's portions are typically smaller than men's portions. That's because women naturally have slower metabolisms, lose weight more slowly, and therefore can't burn up as much food as men can. This is partially a function of the female hormone estrogen, and other hormones, that cause women to retain water. Remember: Everyone is unique, with their own unique metabolism. Whether you're a man or woman, focus on yourself and what you need to do to make progress, and you'll get the body you want.

The best way to control your portions is to weigh and measure your food—*after* cooking it. But if weighing and measuring isn't practical for you, you'll find in the chart below some instructions for estimating portion sizes with foods common to the program. Weigh and measure your foods after cooking them to get the right amounts, since most foods shrink after being cooked.

Food	Portion Size
Protein (fish, poultry breast, or lean meat)	4 oz. = computer mouse, deck of cards, or the palm of your hand; 2 oz. = small packet of matches, or tea bag
Carbohydrates	½ cup of rice = your hand when cupped; 1 cup of rice = your fist; 1 medium potato, sweet potato, or yam = tennis ball
Vegetables and greens	1 cup = your fist
Fruits	½ cup of berries = your hand when cupped

6. Be careful about which tuna you choose. For some body types, I've suggested tuna as a snack. For convenience, it's fine to use canned tuna. Most canned tuna is loaded with salt or sodium, however, and some is packed in oil. Check your grocery store, or better yet your local health food store, for tuna packed in water and labeled "no sodium added"). If you can't find it, buy water-packed tuna and wash it in water to eliminate the sodium. Be aware, too, that certain types of canned tuna, namely white meat tuna, contain high levels of mercury, which can be toxic to health in high amounts. To limit your exposure to mercury, choose canned chunk light tuna instead, or avoid tuna altogether in favor of another type of fish.

Alternatively, cook fresh tuna yourself. It tastes so much better. And you can easily prepare tuna steak in just a few minutes on your grill. After cooking, divide it into the appropriate portions; it will keep in the fridge for days. If you want to add some flavor, try drizzling your tuna with some freshly squeezed lemon juice or a squirt of balsamic vinegar.

7. Always choose the freshest foods possible and prepare them yourself. You want your body to break down the food you feed it as quickly as possible. When you eat food containing preservatives and chemicals, your body chemistry gets sluggish and lethargic, and you stop losing weight. The fresher your food, the better it will taste. If you're used to eating nothing but frozen or canned veggies, you'll be surprised at how good fresh vegetables taste.

You may use canned and frozen vegetables as long as they are labeled "no sodium or sugar added." Keep in mind, however, that you will be much more successful on this makeover program if you stick to fresh vegetables, eaten raw, or lightly steamed.

8. Bake, broil, grill, microwave, or steam your foods—without added oil.

Believe it or not, you don't need any added oil to cook food and vegetables. Simply add a few tablespoons of water to a nonstick pan and quick-cook your egg whites, protein, or vegetables accordingly. Vegetables, in particular, contain their own moisture—another reason why added oil is not necessary. Also, the quality of the newer nonstick cookery these days means there is really no need to grease your pan prior to cooking. Consider this: If you use a teaspoon of butter or oil when you cook every meal, you'd consume an extra 1½ gallons of fat over the course of a year! Another pointer: You may want to stir-fry your vegetables in my special Vegetable Broth (see page 204).

As for vegetable oil spray: Despite the fact that many of these products are labeled "fat-free," the truth of the matter is that they are 100 percent fat. (By law, companies can label their products "fat-free" if the product contains less than a certain amount of fat per serving.) For the six days of this makeover, avoid using vegetable oil sprays to keep your fat intake low. After the six-day period, feel free to use these sprays, but in very small amounts.

9. Be wary of condiments.
Lurking in many condiments are sugar and salt—two bulge makers our diets can do without. Condiments are one of the quickest ways to gain weight! Try enjoying the true taste of fresh food without condiments, or use some of the marinades suggested in appendix A. Do whatever you need to do, within the parameters of your eating plan, to make your food enjoyable. This plays a very key role in your success. And remember: Wholesome, natural, clean-burning food is what helps you lose weight.

10. Avoid all alcoholic beverages during the six days of this program, as well as nonalcoholic beers and wines.
All of these beverages are very high in calories and simple sugars and have the ability to slow down your metabolism and dramatically re-

duce weight loss. What most people don't understand is that alcohol is metabolized in the body like a sugar. That means it ends up being stored as body fat. Alcohol is high in simple sugars, which will slow the weight-loss process. If you want to be successful on the *6-Day Body Makeover,* you must give up alcohol while following the program.

11. Pump the fluids. Drink the following beverages: water (12 eight-ounce glasses of no-sodium-added or distilled water daily), low-sodium/sugar-free soft drinks, and unsweetened tea or coffee.

I know that 12 glasses of water sounds like a lot. But when you drink that amount of water, it keeps your body from retaining any water on its own—which would result in added weight. It also speeds up your overall metabolic rate, and that means even faster weight loss. What I suggest is that you keep five 20-ounce bottles of water close by—at your desk, in your car, wherever and whenever you eat your meals—and make it your goal to drink those five bottles each day. If you're not a big water drinker, add slices of lemon or lime to your water to give it some flavor.

You can still have coffee and/or tea (but without milk, nondairy creamer, or sugar). However, because caffeine dehydrates your body, it does not count toward your allotment of water. In fact, if you are a coffee drinker, you should drink *more* water—in an amount equal to the amount of coffee or tea you drink—to counter the dehydrating effects of caffeine. Herbal teas without caffeine can be counted toward your daily water allotment.

As for diet sodas, most are formulated with sodium, which can cause metabolism-impairing water retention. Avoid club soda as well, since it contains added salt. Diet Rite is one diet soda that does not contain sodium and may be consumed on the *6-Day Body Makeover*—but not in all-you-can-drink amounts. Another alternative is flavored sparkling water for those times you want something bubbly. Check the ingredients first. Some of the flavored sparkling waters contain sodium. Look for low- or no-sodium sparkling waters. Stick to water as your main thirst quencher.

12. Do not eat out at restaurants during the six days of this program. If your diet is ever to get sabotaged, expect it to happen at a restaurant. Some things are just too seductive and tempting when you're trying to lose weight, and restaurants are among them. A lot of restaurant food is battered, fried, creamed, sautéed, or just plain filled with hidden fat, sugar, salt, and other additives that work against your metabolism.

As I've said, the key to the *6-Day Body Makeover* is to eat the exact foods in the right combinations that work with your body to metabolize quickly, so it's vital to avoid all processed foods, as well as added sodium and fat. Frankly, there's just no way to do that at a restaurant. In order for this program to work, you've got to follow it to the letter. Remember, you're losing one whole dress or pant size in only six days, so be religious about all components of this plan during this short period.

Beyond the *6-Day Body Makeover*

This program is a six-day plan—not a long-term approach to weight loss. With its metabolism-tailored food choices, the *6-Day Body Makeover* is carefully designed to help you shed pounds over a six-day period only, so that you aren't demoralized by weeks and weeks of limited food choices. It is permissible to extend the 6-day period to 10 days, if you wish, but no longer than that. After the 6 to 10 days, however, you have the option of switching to my longer-term makeover program, on which you can enjoy a greater selection of foods—as you keep losing pounds and inches at a steady rate. Generally on this program, you can lose up to 30 pounds in six weeks. In chapter 8, you'll find steps on what to do after you've passed the six-day mark.

Nothing is more frustrating than successfully losing pounds and inches, only to gain them all back again. Unlike diets that are virtually impossible to sustain for any extended period of time, my makeover program for further weight loss and maintenance is designed to help you keep your body in shape for life.

Special note if you have a lot of weight to lose (30 or more pounds): I advise clients like you to use the *6-Day Body Makeover* no more than once every six or seven weeks to break a plateau, or to lose those stubborn last 5 pounds. Thus, if you are following my longer-term makeover program, and you find yourself stuck at a plateau, by all means use the *6-Day Body Makeover*. And if you are approaching your goal weight, but want to get there a little faster, it is perfectly fine for you to do that using the *6-Day Body Makeover*.

CHAPTER 4

Customized Eating Plans That Guarantee Rapid Results: The 6-Day Body Makeover *Meals and Menus*

Get ready: You are going to learn how to drop one whole dress or pant size in just six days by using one of five customized meal plans, tailored for your unique body type and metabolism. So if you've been trying hard to knock off pounds (and feeling down on yourself because you can't), these meals and menus have been scientifically designed to work where other methods have failed you. Day by day, you'll witness a remarkable transformation in yourself. You'll see the evidence on your scale and in your mirror as pounds and inches steadily disappear without starvation.

Make sure you have identified your body type before beginning your customized eating plan. Once you've done that, you can start your plan.

You now have the background information that you need to put your plan in action. If you follow your menus as outlined, you'll start experiencing rapid weight loss. What follows are the specific eating plans you should adhere to for the next six days. Each plan is a breeze to follow. Eat exactly what is listed, and you'll be gratified by the way you look and feel—and by how much better your clothes start to fit.

WHEN GRAPEFRUIT AND MEDS DON'T MIX

Grapefruits and grapefruit juice are unique among citrus fruits. Chemicals present in grapefruit and its juice block the action of enzymes that normally break down certain prescription drugs in your body. This can raise blood concentrations over and beyond what the dosage calls for and increase the risk of serious side effects, including heart rhythm disturbances, impaired kidney function, blood pressure changes, and anemia. Typically, the drugs in question are those prescribed to treat heart disease and control blood pressure. If you are taking medication, always read the consumer information sheet that comes with the drug to see what foods, including grapefruit, interfere with the drug's action, or discuss this issue with your doctor. In your case, I advise eating fresh berries instead of grapefruit, or enjoying a quarter of a cantaloupe as a substitute.

Body Type A (Endomorph)

Because you have the slowest metabolism of all the body types—your body may resemble a circle, large and round—yours is the most aggressive eating plan. It is designed to work with your body chemistry in an accelerated fashion that will jump-start your metabolism so that your body will shed pounds and extra body fat very quickly.

Characteristically, many Body Type A's are overweight because of the kinds (and quantities) of proteins and carbohydrates consumed. Given your body chemistry and makeup, your body is particularly sensitive to certain foods, including diet foods, which can have a slowing effect on your metabolism. Many of the foods you are probably eating now are processed and fast foods—all of which signal your body to pack away the calories as fat rather than burn them as fuel. Certain types of carbohydrates, such as simple sugars, processed grains (like breads), and sweet fruits (bananas and other tropical fruits), may cause hikes in your insulin levels. When that happens, insulin tells your body not to release any of the fat it has already stored to burn as calories. It essentially shuts down your metabolism.

As for protein, it does not affect insulin levels, so proteins that are metabolized quickly are not a problem for you. When it comes to protein, the longer it takes to be metabolized and converted into energy, the more that it won't be utilized but will instead be stored as fat. Of the different types of protein, red meat is metabolized the most slowly. This means red meat is *not* the best choice for your body type and may be one of the foods responsible for your sluggish metabolism. Another problem with red meat is that even the leanest cuts have much more fat than other forms of protein. Fat takes longer to metabolize than other types of food. Thus, it will slow your metabolism even further.

Foods That Trigger Weight Loss for Body Type A

As a Body Type A, what you must do is replace the carbohydrates and proteins that are slowing your metabolism with greater quantities of those types of foods that will speed it up. Not all carbohydrates act the same way in the body. You need to concentrate on certain types of natural carbohydrates because they are converted to fuel more readily for your body type. For example, your body will have much better results with potatoes, sweet potatoes, yams, and low-sugar fruits such as berries and grapefruit. These foods cause less of an insulin response—and therefore less fat storage.

As for protein, you will see much better results with fish and with boneless, skinless chicken or turkey breasts than with red meat. Most people with your body type will experience rapid results with fish because it is metabolized very quickly and really stokes up your body's fat-burning furnace. Thus, your eating plan calls for quite a bit of fast-metabolizing fish. As you will see in the permissible foods list I've created for you, there is a huge variety of fish from which you can choose.

Special note: If you don't care for the taste of fish, I'd like you to at least try some form of it as one of your protein sources. You will always see much better results when you eat fish because it's metabolized very quickly and will really stoke up your body's fat-burning furnace. If you absolutely can't stomach fish, you'll also get good results with lean chicken or turkey.

Body Type A Makeover: Permissible Foods List

Proteins		Carbohydrates		Vegetables	Greens
Poultry	**Fish**	**Starches**	**Fruits**		
Egg whites	Cod	Potato	Blackberries	Alfalfa	Arugula
Chicken	Flounder	Sweet potato	Blueberries	sprouts	Beet greens
breast,	Grouper	Yam	Boysenberries	Asparagus	Collard
skin	Haddock		Grapefruit	Broccoli	greens
removed	Halibut		Raspberries	Brussels	Dandelion
Chicken	Monkfish		Strawberries	sprouts	greens
breast,	Orange			Cabbage	Endive
ground	roughy			Cauliflower	Kale
Turkey	Perch			Celery	Lettuce, all
breast,	Pollack			Cucumber	varieties
skin	Red snapper			Eggplant	Mustard
removed	Shark			Garlic	greens
Turkey	Sole			Green beans	Parsley
breast,	Tilapia			Mushrooms	Spinach
ground	Trout			Okra	Swiss
	Tuna			Onions	chard
	(fresh or			Pea pods	Turnip
	no-sodium-			Peppers, all	greens
	added			varieties	Watercress
	canned)			Scallions	
	Whitefish			Summer	
				squash, all	
				varieties	
				Zucchini	

The *6-Day Body Makeover* Eating Plan for Body Type A

The Body Type A Eating Plan specifies exactly what you should eat (and in what quantities) for the next six days. I've provided a template for you, to show you the basics of a typical day on the Body Type A Eating Plan. In the section that follows this template, you'll find a day-by-day eating plan for Body Type A. This plan tells you exactly what to eat on each of the six days and is designed to remove all the guesswork from your meal planning. The recipes suggested here can be found in appendix A.

Very important:

- Do not deviate from the permissible foods that were listed previously or are listed in your menus.

- Follow your eating plan exactly with regard to the food suggestions. *Make no substitutions* for the suggested food unless you're substituting lean poultry for fish.

- If you don't like the suggested recipe or would prefer a different method of preparation, check appendix A for an alternative recipe that suits your body type.

- Pay strict attention to portion sizes.

- Do not use oil, mayonnaise, salad dressings (except those in appendix A), butter, margarine, vegetable oil spray, or any other added oils or fats.

- Never skip any meals, except for the optional PM snack.

- Drink 100 ounces (approximately twelve 8-ounce glasses) of water daily.

A Typical Day — Eating Plan Template for Body Type A

BREAKFAST

Men: 4 oz. turkey sausage and ½ grapefruit (or ½ cup mixed berries)

Women: 3 oz. turkey sausage and ½ grapefruit (or ½ cup mixed berries)

MIDMORNING SNACK

Men: 4 oz. fresh tuna or no-sodium-added canned tuna and 1 cup greens (any type)

Women: 3 oz. fresh tuna or no-sodium-added canned tuna and 1 cup greens (any type)

LUNCH

Men: 4 oz. fish, 1 medium potato or yam, and 1 cup greens (any type)

Women: 2 oz. fish, ½ medium baked potato or yam, and 1 cup greens (any type)

MIDAFTERNOON SNACK

Men: 4 oz. fresh tuna or no-sodium-added canned tuna and 1 cup greens (any type)

Women: 3 oz. fresh tuna or no-sodium-added canned tuna and 1 cup greens (any type)

DINNER

Men: 4 oz. fish, 1 medium baked potato or yam, and 1 cup greens

Women: 2 oz. fish, ½ medium baked potato or yam, and 1 cup greens

PM SNACK (OPTIONAL)

Men: 2 oz. chicken breast and 1 cup greens

Women: 2 oz. chicken breast and 1 cup greens

Day-by-Day Eating Plan for Body Type A (with Recipes)

BREAKFAST

Men

1 serving Turkey Sausage Patties
(page 192)

½ grapefruit

Women

½ serving Turkey Sausage Patties
(page 192)

½ grapefruit

MIDMORNING SNACK

Men

4 oz. fresh Grilled Tuna Steak (page 188)
or no-sodium-added canned tuna

1 cup greens (any type) with Cucumber
Vinaigrette (page 213)

Women

3 oz. fresh Grilled Tuna Steak (page 188)
or no-sodium-added canned tuna

1 cup greens (any type) with Cucumber
Vinaigrette (page 213)

LUNCH

Men

4 oz. Grilled Red Snapper with Fennel
(page 186) or 4 oz. fish

1 medium yam or baked potato

1 cup greens (any type) with Cucumber
Vinaigrette (page 213)

Women

2 oz. Grilled Red Snapper with Fennel
(page 186) or 2 oz. fish

½ medium yam or baked potato

1 cup greens (any type) with Cucumber
Vinaigrette (page 213)

MIDAFTERNOON SNACK

Men

4 oz. fresh tuna or no-sodium-added
canned tuna

1 cup greens (any type)

Women

3 oz. fresh tuna or no-sodium-added
canned tuna

1 cup greens (any type)

SUNDAY

DINNER

Men	Women
4 oz. fish	2 oz. fish
1 serving Perfect Mashed Potatoes (page 210)	½ serving Perfect Mashed Potatoes (page 210)
1 cup greens (any type) with Cucumber Vinaigrette (page 213)	1 cup greens (any type) with Cucumber Vinaigrette (page 213)

PM SNACK (OPTIONAL)

Men	Women
2 oz. chicken breast	2 oz. chicken breast
1 cup greens (any type)	1 cup greens (any type)

MONDAY

BREAKFAST

Men	Women
1 serving Turkey Sausage Patties (page 192)	½ serving Turkey Sausage Patties (page 192)
½ cup blueberries or raspberries	½ cup blueberries or raspberries

MIDMORNING SNACK

Men	Women
4 oz. no-sodium-added canned tuna	3 oz. no-sodium-added canned tuna
1 cup greens (any type) with Cucumber Vinaigrette (page 213)	1 cup greens (any type) with Cucumber Vinaigrette (page 213)

LUNCH

Men	Women
4 oz. Steam-Poached Fish Fillets (page 190) or 4 oz. fish	2 oz. Steam-Poached Fish Fillets (page 190) or 2 oz. fish
1 serving Oven-Baked French Fries (page 209)	½ serving Oven-Baked French Fries (page 209)
1 cup greens (any type)	1 cup greens (any type)

MIDAFTERNOON SNACK

Men

4 oz. fresh tuna or no-sodium-added
    canned tuna

1 cup greens (any type)

Women

3 oz. fresh tuna or no-sodium-added
    canned tuna

1 cup greens (any type)

DINNER

Men

4 oz. fish

1 serving Perfect Mashed Potatoes
    (page 210)

1 cup asparagus or other green vegetable

Women

2 oz. fish

½ serving Perfect Mashed Potatoes
    (page 210)

1 cup asparagus or other green vegetable

PM SNACK (OPTIONAL)

Men

2 oz. chicken breast

1 cup greens (any type)

Women

2 oz. chicken breast

1 cup greens (any type)

BREAKFAST

Men

1 serving Turkey Sausage Patties
    (page 192)

Broiled Cinnamon Grapefruit (page 221)

Women

½ serving Turkey Sausage Patties
    (page 192)

Broiled Cinnamon Grapefruit (page 221)

MIDMORNING SNACK

Men

4 oz. fresh Grilled Tuna Steak (page 188)
    or no-sodium-added canned tuna

1 cup Green Bean Salad (page 216) or
    1 cup greens (any type) with Cucumber Vinaigrette (page 213)

Women

3 oz. fresh Grilled Tuna Steak (page 188)
    or no-sodium-added canned tuna

1 cup Green Bean Salad (page 216) or
    1 cup greens (any type) with Cucumber Vinaigrette (page 213)

LUNCH

Men	Women
4 oz. Fish and Vegetable Kebabs (page 189) or 4 oz. fish	2 oz. Fish and Vegetable Kebabs (page 189) or 4 oz. fish
One 5–6 oz. potato or yam	One 3–4 oz. potato or yam
1 cup mixed vegetables	1 cup mixed vegetables

MIDAFTERNOON SNACK

Men	Women
4 oz. fresh tuna or no-sodium-added canned tuna	3 oz. fresh tuna or no-sodium-added canned tuna
1 cup greens (any type)	1 cup greens (any type)

DINNER

Men	Women
4 oz. fish	2 oz. fish
1 serving Oven-Baked French Fries (page 209)	½ serving Oven-Baked French Fries (page 209)
1 cup broccoli, cauliflower, spinach, or other vegetable	1 cup broccoli, cauliflower, spinach, or other vegetable

PM SNACK (OPTIONAL)

Men	Women
2 oz. chicken breast	2 oz. chicken breast
1 cup greens (any type)	1 cup greens (any type)

BREAKFAST

Men	Women
1 serving Turkey Sausage Patties (page 192)	½ serving Turkey Sausage Patties (page 192)
½ cup strawberries or other berries in season	½ cup strawberries or other berries in season

TUESDAY

WEDNESDAY

MIDMORNING SNACK

Men

4 oz. fresh Grilled Tuna Steak (page 188)
   or no-sodium-added canned tuna

1 cup greens (any type) with Cucumber
   Vinaigrette (page 213)

Women

3 oz. fresh Grilled Tuna Steak (page 188)
   or no-sodium-added canned tuna

1 cup greens (any type) with Cucumber
   Vinaigrette (page 213)

LUNCH

Men

4 oz. fish

One 5–6 oz. potato or yam

1 cup Summer Squash Medley (page 208)

Women

2 oz. fish

One 3–4 oz. baked potato or yam

1 cup Summer Squash Medley (page 208)

MIDAFTERNOON SNACK

Men

4 oz. fresh tuna or no-sodium-added
   canned tuna

1 cup greens (any type)

Women

3 oz. fresh tuna or no-sodium-added
   canned tuna

1 cup greens (any type)

DINNER

Men

4 oz. Fish and Vegetable Kebabs
   (page 189)

1 serving Perfect Mashed Potatoes
   (page 210)

Women

2 oz. Fish and Vegetable Kebabs
   (page 189)

½ serving Perfect Mashed Potatoes
   (page 210)

PM SNACK (OPTIONAL)

Men

2 oz. chicken breast

1 cup greens (any type)

Women

2 oz. chicken breast

1 cup greens (any type)

BREAKFAST

Men

1 serving Turkey Sausage Patties
(page 192)

½ grapefruit (or ½ cup mixed berries)

Women

½ serving Turkey Sausage Patties
(page 192)

½ grapefruit (or ½ cup mixed berries)

MIDMORNING SNACK

Men

4 oz. no-sodium-added canned tuna

1 cup greens (any type) with Cucumber
Vinaigrette (page 213)

Women

3 oz. no-sodium-added canned tuna

1 cup greens (any type) with Cucumber
Vinaigrette (page 213)

LUNCH

Men

1 serving Ceviche Salad (page 191)
served over 1 cup shredded lettuce

1 serving Oven-Baked French Fries
(page 209) or one 5–6 oz. potato or yam

Women

½ serving Ceviche Salad (page 191)
served over 1 cup shredded lettuce

½ serving Oven-Baked French Fries
(page 209) or one 3–4 oz. potato or yam

MIDAFTERNOON SNACK

Men

4 oz. fresh tuna or no-sodium-added
canned tuna

1 cup greens (any type)

Women

3 oz. fresh tuna or no-sodium-added
canned tuna

1 cup greens (any type)

DINNER

Men

4 oz. fish

1 cup Spicy Asparagus (page 208) or
1 cup greens (any type) or mixed
vegetables

1 serving Perfect Mashed Potatoes
(page 210) or one 5–6 oz. baked
potato or yam

Women

2 oz. fish

1 cup Spicy Asparagus (page 208) or
1 cup greens (any type) or mixed
vegetables

½ serving Perfect Mashed Potatoes
(page 210) or one 3–4 oz. baked
potato or yam

THURSDAY

PM SNACK (OPTIONAL)

Men

2 oz. chicken breast

1 cup greens (any type)

Women

2 oz. chicken breast

1 cup greens (any type)

BREAKFAST

Men

1 serving Turkey Sausage Patties
(page 192)

½ grapefruit

Women

½ serving Turkey Sausage Patties
(page 192)

½ grapefruit

MIDMORNING SNACK

Men

4 oz. fresh Grilled Tuna Steak (page 188)
or no-sodium-added canned tuna

1 cup greens (any type) with Cucumber
Vinaigrette (page 213)

Women

3 oz. fresh Grilled Tuna Steak (page 188)
or no-sodium-added canned tuna

1 cup greens (any type) with Cucumber
Vinaigrette (page 213)

LUNCH

Men

4 oz. fish

1 serving Oven-Baked French Fries
(page 209) or one 5–6 oz. baked potato
or yam

1 cup greens (any type) with Cucumber
Vinaigrette (page 213)

Women

2 oz. fish

½ serving Oven-Baked French Fries
(page 209) or one 3–4 oz. baked potato
or yam

1 cup greens (any type) with Cucumber
Vinaigrette (page 213)

MIDAFTERNOON SNACK

Men

4 oz. fresh tuna or no-sodium-added
   canned tuna

1 cup greens (any type)

Women

3 oz. fresh tuna or no-sodium-added
   canned tuna

1 cup greens (any type)

DINNER

Men

1 serving Herb-Crusted Fish (page 191)
   or 4 oz. fish

1 serving Perfect Mashed Potatoes
   (page 210) or one 5–6 oz. baked potato
   or yam

1 cup greens (any type) or 1 cup other
   vegetables

Women

½ serving Herb-Crusted Fish (page 191)
   or 2 oz. fish

½ serving Perfect Mashed Potatoes
   (page 210) or one 3–4 oz. baked potato
   or yam

1 cup greens (any type) or 1 cup other
   vegetables

PM SNACK (OPTIONAL)

Men

2 oz. chicken breast

1 cup greens (any type)

Women

2 oz. chicken breast

1 cup greens (any type)

FRIDAY

Body Type B (Endo-Meso)

Despite the advantage of adequate muscle tissue, Body Type B's, your body may resemble a triangle, with body fat concentrated in your stomach, hips, thighs, and buttocks, and you have a metabolism that isn't fast enough to keep the weight off. As with most body types, the choice of too many processed and fast foods, plus slow-metabolizing proteins, contributes to a sluggish metabolic rate. As a Body Type B, you must focus on complex carbohydrates that are converted less quickly to sugar so that you don't further slow your metabolism. You'll also need to carefully balance the ratio of carbs to certain proteins. Particularly with your body chemistry, eating too many of the wrong types of carbs, without some other type of food to slow down their conversion to sugar, can essentially grind your metabolism to a halt and make it impossible to lose weight.

Body Type B's generally have plenty of muscle on their bodies—sometimes too much. Women, in particular, may have very large, muscular thighs and buttocks—and they don't want to get any bigger in any way. If you are a Body Type B, you probably want to reduce your body size all over and replace large overly muscular parts of your body with longer, leaner, more slenderized muscles. Because red meat can cause you to bulk up, you will have more success concentrating on other sources of protein such as fish, chicken breasts, and turkey breasts.

Foods That Trigger Weight Loss for Body Type B

The key to accelerating your metabolism for quick weight loss over the next six days is to very carefully regulate the type and quantity of complex carbs and proteins you eat. Because you do have a slow metabolism, your eating plan includes slightly fewer carbohydrates than some of the other body types (which have somewhat faster metabolisms, and aren't as sensitive to insulin spikes as you are). Basically, your body will respond best to natural grains such as brown rice (which supplies roughly three times as much fiber as is found in instant white rice, plus essential nutrients such as folate, riboflavin, iron, and magnesium) and to low-sugar fruits such as grapefruit and berries. Since these fruits have less sugar, there is less risk of elevating your insulin level and slowing down your weight loss. Sweeter fruits like cherries, oranges, or watermelon will further slow down your already sluggish metabolism, so be sure to avoid those while following this program.

Body Type B Makeover: Permissible Foods List

Proteins		Carbohydrates		Vegetables	Greens
Poultry	**Fish**	***Starches**	**Fruits**		
Egg whites	Cod	Brown rice	Blackberries	Alfalfa sprouts	Arugula
Chicken	Flounder	Long-grain	Blueberries	Asparagus	Beet
breast,	Grouper	rice	Boysenberries	Broccoli	greens
skin	Haddock	White rice,	Grapefruit	Brussels sprouts	Collard
removed	Halibut	or wild	Raspberries	Cabbage	greens
Chicken	Monkfish	rice	Strawberries	Cauliflower	Dandelion
breast,	Orange			Celery	greens
ground	roughy			Cucumber	Endive
Turkey	Perch			Eggplant	Kale
breast,	Pollack			Garlic	Lettuce, all
skin	Red snapper			Green beans	varieties
removed	Shark			Mushrooms	Mustard
Turkey	Sole			Okra	greens
breast,	Tilapia			Onions	Parsley
ground	Trout			Pea pods	Spinach
	Tuna			Peppers, all	Swiss
	(fresh or			varieties	chard
	no-sodium-			Scallions	Turnip
	added			Summer	greens
	canned)			squash, all	Watercress
	Whitefish			varieties	
				Zucchini	

These varieties of rice cause less of an elevation in blood sugar than instant white rice does and are the preferred choices for rice on your customized eating plan.

The *6-Day Body Makeover* Eating Plan for Body Type B

The Body Type B Eating Plan specifies exactly what you should eat (and in what quantities) for the next six days. I've provided a template for you, to show you the basics of a typical day on the Body Type B Eating Plan. In the section that follows this template, you'll find a day-by-day eating plan for Body Type B. This plan tells you exactly what to eat on each of the six days and is designed to remove all the guesswork from your meal planning. The recipes suggested here can be found in appendix A.

Very important:

- Do not deviate from the permissible foods that were listed previously or are listed in your menus.

- Follow your eating plan exactly with regard to the food suggestions. *Make no substitutions* for the suggested food unless you're substituting lean poultry for fish.

- If you don't like the suggested recipe or would prefer a different method of preparation, check appendix A for an alternative recipe that suits your body type.

- Pay strict attention to portion sizes.

- Do not use oil, mayonnaise, salad dressings (except those in appendix A), butter, margarine, vegetable oil spray, or any other added oils or fats.

- Never skip any meals, except for the optional PM snack.

- Drink 100 ounces (approximately twelve 8-ounce glasses) of water daily.

A Typical Day — Eating Plan Template for Body Type B

BREAKFAST

Men: 4 scrambled egg whites (or 4 oz. turkey sausage) and ½ grapefruit (or ½ cup mixed berries)

Women: 3 scrambled egg whites (or 3 oz. turkey sausage) and ½ grapefruit (or ½ cup mixed berries)

MIDMORNING SNACK

Men: 4 oz. turkey breast and 1 cup greens (any type)

Women: 3 oz. turkey breast and 1 cup greens (any type)

LUNCH

Men: 4 oz. chicken breast, 1 cup rice, and 1 cup mixed vegetables

Women: 2 oz. chicken breast, ½ cup rice, and 1 cup mixed vegetables

MIDAFTERNOON SNACK

Men: 4 oz. fresh tuna or no-sodium-added canned tuna and 1 cup greens (any type)

Women: 3 oz. fresh tuna or no-sodium-added canned tuna and 1 cup greens (any type)

DINNER

Men: 4 oz. chicken breast, 1 cup rice, and 1 cup mixed vegetables

Women: 2 oz. chicken breast, ½ cup rice, and 1 cup mixed vegetables

PM SNACK (OPTIONAL)

Men: ½ grapefruit (or ½ cup mixed berries)

Women: ½ grapefruit (or ½ cup mixed berries)

Day-by-Day Eating Plan for Body Type B (with Recipes)

BREAKFAST

Men	*Women*
4 scrambled egg whites or 1 serving Turkey Sausage Patties (page 192)	3 scrambled egg whites or ½ serving Turkey Sausage Patties (page 192)
½ grapefruit (or ½ cup mixed berries)	½ grapefruit (or ½ cup mixed berries)

MIDMORNING SNACK

Men	*Women*
4 oz. turkey breast (baked plain or in Indian Marinade—page 184)	3 oz. turkey breast (baked plain or in Indian Marinade—page 184)
1 cup greens (any type) with Cucumber Vinaigrette (page 213)	1 cup greens (any type) with Cucumber Vinaigrette (page 213)

SUNDAY

LUNCH

Men	Women
4 oz. chicken breast	2 oz. chicken breast
1 cup Spanish Rice (page 211)	½ cup Spanish Rice (page 211)
1 cup mixed vegetables	1 cup mixed vegetables

MIDAFTERNOON SNACK

Men	Women
4 oz. fresh tuna or no-sodium-added canned tuna	3 oz. fresh tuna or no-sodium-added canned tuna
1 cup greens (any type)	1 cup greens (any type)

DINNER

Men	Women
4 oz. Roast Chicken with Vegetables (page 194)	2 oz. Roast Chicken with Vegetables (page 194)
1 cup rice	½ cup rice

PM SNACK (OPTIONAL)

Men	Women
½ grapefruit (or ½ cup mixed berries)	½ grapefruit (or ½ cup mixed berries)

BREAKFAST

Men	Women
4 scrambled egg whites or 1 serving Turkey Sausage Patties (page 192)	3 scrambled egg whites or ½ serving Turkey Sausage Patties (page 192)
½ Broiled Cinnamon Grapefruit (page 221)	½ Broiled Cinnamon Grapefruit (page 221)

MIDMORNING SNACK

Men	Women
4 oz. turkey breast	3 oz. turkey breast
1 cup greens (any type) with Cucumber Vinaigrette (page 213)	1 cup greens (any type) with Cucumber Vinaigrette (page 213)

LUNCH

Men

1 serving Orange and Garlic Chicken
 (page 193) or 4 oz. chicken breast

1 cup brown rice

1 cup mixed vegetables

Women

½ serving Orange and Garlic Chicken
 (page 193) or 2 oz. chicken breast

½ cup brown rice

1 cup mixed vegetables

MIDAFTERNOON SNACK

Men

4 oz. fresh tuna or no-sodium-added
 canned tuna

1 cup greens (any type)

Women

3 oz. fresh tuna or no-sodium-added
 canned tuna

1 cup greens (any type)

DINNER

Men

1 serving Chicken and Asparagus Stir-Fry
 (page 196) or 4 oz. chicken

1 cup brown rice

Women

½ serving Chicken and Asparagus
 Stir-Fry (page 196) or 2 oz. chicken

½ cup brown rice

PM SNACK (OPTIONAL)

Men

½ cup mixed berries

Women

½ cup mixed berries

BREAKFAST

Men

1 serving Egg White Meringue Cookies
 (page 221, made with 4 egg whites)
 or 1 serving Turkey Sausage Patties
 (page 192)

½ cup sliced strawberries

Women

1 serving Egg White Meringue Cookies
 (page 221, made with 3 egg whites) or
 ½ serving Turkey Sausage Patties
 (page 192)

½ cup sliced strawberries

MONDAY

TUESDAY

MIDMORNING SNACK

Men

4 oz. turkey breast

1 cup mixed vegetables

Women

3 oz. turkey breast

1 cup mixed vegetables

LUNCH

Men

4 oz. chicken breast

1 cup brown rice

1 serving Gazpacho (page 207) or 1 cup
   mixed vegetables

Women

2 oz. chicken breast

½ cup brown rice

1 serving Gazpacho (page 207) or 1 cup
   mixed vegetables

MIDAFTERNOON SNACK

Men

4 oz. fresh tuna or no-sodium-added
   canned tuna

1 cup greens (any type)

Women

3 oz. fresh tuna or no-sodium-added
   canned tuna

1 cup greens (any type)

DINNER

Men

1 serving Jamaican Chicken (page 200) or
   4 oz. chicken

1 cup brown rice

1 cup asparagus or other vegetable

Women

½ serving Jamaican Chicken (page 200)
   or 2 oz. chicken

½ cup brown rice

1 cup asparagus or other vegetable

PM SNACK (OPTIONAL)

Men

½ grapefruit (or ½ cup mixed berries)

Women

½ grapefruit (or ½ cup mixed berries)

BREAKFAST

Men	Women
1 serving Turkey Sausage Patties (page 192)	½ serving Turkey Sausage Patties (page 192)
½ cup blueberries or other berries in season	½ cup blueberries or other berries in season

MIDMORNING SNACK

Men	Women
4 oz. turkey breast	3 oz. turkey breast
1 cup greens (any type) with Cucumber Vinaigrette (page 213)	1 cup greens (any type) with Cucumber Vinaigrette (page 213)

LUNCH

Men	Women
4 oz. chicken breast	2 oz. chicken breast
1 cup Spanish Rice (page 211)	½ cup Spanish Rice (page 211)
1 cup mixed vegetables	1 cup mixed vegetables

MIDAFTERNOON SNACK

Men	Women
4 oz. fresh tuna or no-sodium-added canned tuna	3 oz. fresh tuna or no-sodium-added canned tuna
1 cup greens (any type)	1 cup greens (any type)

DINNER

Men	Women
1 serving Spicy Chicken (page 198) or 4 oz. chicken breast	½ serving Spicy Chicken (page 198) or 2 oz. chicken breast
1 cup rice	½ cup rice
1 cup mixed green salad with lemon juice or balsamic vinegar	1 cup mixed green salad with lemon juice or balsamic vinegar

WEDNESDAY

PM SNACK (OPTIONAL)

Men

½ Broiled Cinnamon Grapefruit
 (page 221)

Women

½ Broiled Cinnamon Grapefruit
 (page 221)

BREAKFAST

Men

4 scrambled egg whites or 1 serving
 Turkey Sausage Patties (page 192)

½ grapefruit

Women

3 scrambled egg whites or ½ serving
 Turkey Sausage Patties (page 192)

½ grapefruit

MIDMORNING SNACK

Men

4 oz. turkey breast (baked plain or in
 Cuban Lime Marinade—page 184)

1 cup greens (any type) with Cucumber
 Vinaigrette (page 213)

Women

3 oz. turkey breast (baked plain or in
 Cuban Lime Marinade—page 184)

1 cup greens (any type) with Cucumber
 Vinaigrette (page 213)

LUNCH

Men

4 oz. chicken breast

1 cup rice

1 cup Grilled Vegetables (page 205)

Women

2 oz. chicken breast

½ cup rice

1 cup Grilled Vegetables (page 205)

MIDAFTERNOON SNACK

Men

4 oz. fresh tuna or no-sodium-added
 canned tuna

1 cup greens (any type)

Women

3 oz. fresh tuna or no-sodium-added
 canned tuna

1 cup greens (any type)

DINNER

THURSDAY

Men	Women
4 oz. Roast Chicken with Vegetables (page 194)	2 oz. Roast Chicken with Vegetables (page 194)
1 cup rice	½ cup rice
1 cup mixed green salad with lemon juice or balsamic vinegar	1 cup mixed green salad with lemon juice or balsamic vinegar

PM SNACK (OPTIONAL)

Men	Women
½ cup mixed berries	½ cup mixed berries

BREAKFAST

FRIDAY

Men	Women
4 scrambled egg whites or 1 serving Turkey Sausage Patties (page 192)	3 scrambled egg whites or ½ serving Turkey Sausage Patties (page 192)
½ grapefruit (or ½ cup mixed berries)	½ grapefruit (or ½ cup mixed berries)

MIDMORNING SNACK

Men	Women
4 oz. turkey breast	3 oz. turkey breast
1 cup greens (any type) with Cucumber Vinaigrette (page 213)	1 cup greens (any type) with Cucumber Vinaigrette (page 213)

LUNCH

Men	Women
1 serving Poached Chicken (page 197) or 4 oz. chicken breast	½ serving Poached Chicken (page 197) or 2 oz. chicken breast
1 cup Spanish Rice (page 211)	½ cup Spanish Rice (page 211)
1 cup broccoli or other vegetable	1 cup broccoli or other vegetable

MIDAFTERNOON SNACK

Men

4 oz. fresh tuna or no-sodium-added
  canned tuna

1 cup greens (any type)

Women

3 oz. fresh tuna or no-sodium-added
  canned tuna

1 cup greens (any type)

DINNER

Men

2 Stuffed Peppers (page 195) or 4 oz.
  chicken breast with 1 cup mixed
  vegetables and 1 cup rice

Women

1 Stuffed Pepper (page 195) or 2 oz.
  chicken breast with 1 cup mixed
  vegetables and ½ cup rice

PM SNACK (OPTIONAL)

Men

½ grapefruit (or ½ cup mixed berries)

Women

½ grapefruit (or ½ cup mixed berries)

Body Type C (Meso-Endo)

As a Body Type C—your body may resemble a rectangle, a thick-bodied frame and roughly the same width at shoulders, waist, and hips—your metabolism isn't quite as slow as some of the other body types because you generally have plenty of metabolically active muscle. More than other body types, you can eat slightly more carbohydrates, although you must be careful about the types and quantities you do eat. Your body will generally react better to complex carbohydrates since simple carbs like sweet fruits, simple sugars, and processed grains will slow your metabolism down even further. And, as with all body types, make sure you always eat a carbohydrate with a protein to prevent your blood sugar and insulin levels from spiking—a reaction that can shut down your metabolism and its ability to burn fat. If you happen to be a Body Type C, you can handle nearly all the vegetables you desire, since they have very few calories and almost no effect on metabolism.

Generally, a Body Type C wants to reduce body size all over and replace large, overly muscular parts of the body with longer, leaner muscle. Your plan is specially designed to fire up your metabolic rate, but without bulking you up. If you weight train, that means no red meat as protein, since you run the risk of adding too much muscle. You'll get better results with chicken or fish as your protein sources; both metabolize quickly to further accelerate your slower-than-normal metabolism.

Body Type C Makeover: Permissible Foods List

Proteins		Carbohydrates		Vegetables	Greens
Poultry	**Fish**	**Starches**	**Fruits**		
Egg whites	Cod	Brown rice	Blackberries	Alfalfa	Arugula
Chicken	Flounder	Long-grain	Blueberries	sprouts	Beet greens
breast,	Grouper	rice	Boysenberries	Asparagus	Collard
skin	Haddock	Wild rice	Grapefruit	Broccoli	greens
removed	Halibut		Raspberries	Brussels	Dandelion
Chicken	Monkfish		Strawberries	sprouts	greens
breast,	Orange			Cabbage	Endive
ground	roughy			Cauliflower	Kale

Proteins				Vegetables	Greens
Poultry	**Fish**				
Turkey	Perch			Celery	Lettuce, all
breast,	Pollack			Cucumber	varieties
skin	Red snapper			Eggplant	Mustard
removed	Shark			Garlic	greens
Turkey	Sole			Green beans	Parsley
breast,	Tilapia			Mushrooms	Spinach
ground	Trout			Okra	Swiss
	Tuna			Onions	chard
	(fresh or			Pea pods	Turnip
	no-			Peppers, all	greens
	sodium-			varieties	Watercress
	added			Scallions	
	canned)			Summer	
	Whitefish			squash, all	
				varieties	
				Zucchini	

The *6-Day Body Makeover* Eating Plan for Body Type C

The Body Type C Eating Plan specifies exactly what you should eat (and in what quantities) for the next six days. I've provided a template for you, to show you the basics of a typical day on the Body Type C Eating Plan. In the section that follows this template, you'll find a day-by-day eating plan for Body Type C. This plan tells you exactly what to eat on each of the six days and is designed to remove all the guesswork from your meal planning. The recipes suggested here can be found in appendix A.

Very important:

- Do not deviate from the permissible foods that were listed previously or are listed in your menus.

- Follow your eating plan exactly with regard to the food suggestions. *Make no substitutions* for the suggested food unless you're substituting lean poultry for fish.
- If you don't like the suggested recipe or would prefer a different method of preparation, check appendix A for an alternative recipe that suits your body type.
- Pay strict attention to portion sizes.
- Do not use oil, mayonnaise, salad dressings (except those in appendix A), butter, margarine, vegetable oil spray, or any other added oils or fats.
- Never skip any meals, except for the optional PM snack.
- Drink 100 ounces (approximately twelve 8-ounce glasses) of water daily.

A Typical Day—Eating Plan Template for Body Type C

BREAKFAST

Men: 4 scrambled egg whites (or 4 oz. turkey sausage) and ½ grapefruit (or ½ cup mixed berries)

Women: 3 scrambled egg whites (or 3 oz. turkey sausage) and ½ grapefruit (or ½ cup mixed berries)

MIDMORNING SNACK

Men: 4 oz. turkey breast and 1 to 2 cups greens (any type)

Women: 3 oz. turkey breast and 1 to 2 cups greens (any type)

LUNCH

Men: 4 oz. chicken breast, 1 cup rice, and 1 to 2 cups mixed vegetables

Women: 2 oz. chicken breast, ½ cup rice, and 1 to 2 cups mixed vegetables

MIDAFTERNOON SNACK

Men: 4 oz. fresh tuna or no-sodium-added canned tuna and 1 to 2 cups greens (any type)

Women: 3 oz. fresh tuna or no-sodium-added canned tuna and 1 to 2 cups greens (any type)

DINNER

Men: 4 oz. chicken breast, 1 cup rice, and 1 to 2 cups mixed vegetables

Women: 2 oz. baked chicken breast, ½ cup rice, and 1 to 2 cups mixed vegetables

PM SNACK (OPTIONAL)

Men: 1 grapefruit (or 1 cup mixed berries)

Women: 1 grapefruit (or 1 cup mixed berries)

Day-by-Day Eating Plan for Body Type C (with Recipes)

BREAKFAST

Men	Women
4 scrambled egg whites or 1 serving Turkey Sausage Patties (page 192)	3 scrambled egg whites or ½ serving Turkey Sausage Patties (page 192)
½ grapefruit or ½ cup mixed berries	½ grapefruit or ½ cup mixed berries

MIDMORNING SNACK

Men	Women
4 oz. baked turkey breast	2 oz. baked turkey breast
1 to 2 cups greens (any type) with Cucumber Vinaigrette (page 213)	1 to 2 cups greens (any type) with Cucumber Vinaigrette (page 213)

LUNCH

Men	Women
1 serving Lemon Oregano Chicken (page 197) or 4 oz. baked chicken breast	½ serving Lemon Oregano Chicken (page 197) or 2 oz. baked chicken breast
1 cup rice	½ cup rice
1 to 2 cups mixed vegetables	1 to 2 cups mixed vegetables

MIDAFTERNOON SNACK

Men

4 oz. fresh tuna or no-sodium-added
   canned tuna

1 to 2 cups greens (any type) with
   Cucumber Vinaigrette (page 213)

Women

3 oz. fresh tuna or no-sodium-added
   canned tuna

1 to 2 cups greens (any type) with
   Cucumber Vinaigrette (page 213)

DINNER

Men

1 serving Orange and Garlic Chicken
   (page 193) or 4 oz. baked chicken
   breast

1 cup brown rice

1 to 2 cups Summer Squash Medley
   (page 208) or 1 to 2 cups mixed
   vegetables

Women

½ serving Orange and Garlic Chicken
   (page 193) or 2 oz. baked chicken
   breast

½ cup brown rice

1 to 2 cups Summer Squash Medley
   (page 208) or 1 to 2 cups mixed
   vegetables

PM SNACK (OPTIONAL)

Men

1 grapefruit (or 1 cup mixed berries)

Women

1 grapefruit (or 1 cup mixed berries)

BREAKFAST

Men

4 scrambled egg whites or 1 serving
   Turkey Sausage Patties (page 192)

½ Broiled Cinnamon Grapefruit
   (page 221)

Women

3 scrambled egg whites or ½ serving
   Turkey Sausage Patties (page 192)

½ Broiled Cinnamon Grapefruit
   (page 221)

MIDMORNING SNACK

Men

4 oz. baked turkey breast

1 to 2 cups greens (any type) with
   Cucumber Vinaigrette (page 213)

Women

3 oz. baked turkey breast

1 to 2 cups greens (any type) with
   Cucumber Vinaigrette (page 213)

SUNDAY

MONDAY

LUNCH

Men

1 serving Roast Chicken with Vegetables
(page 194) or 4 oz. baked chicken
breast
1 cup rice
1 to 2 cups mixed vegetables

Women

½ serving Roast Chicken with Vegetables
(page 194) or 2 oz. baked chicken
breast
½ cup rice
1 to 2 cups mixed vegetables

MIDAFTERNOON SNACK

Men

4 oz. fresh tuna or no-sodium-added
canned tuna
1 to 2 cups greens (any type) with
Cucumber Vinaigrette (page 213)

Women

3 oz. fresh tuna or no-sodium-added
canned tuna
1 to 2 cups greens (any type) with
Cucumber Vinaigrette (page 213)

DINNER

Men

2 Stuffed Peppers (page 195) or 4 oz.
baked chicken breast with 1 cup brown
rice and 1 to 2 cups mixed vegetables

Women

1 Stuffed Pepper (page 195) or 2 oz. baked
chicken breast with ½ cup brown rice
and 1 to 2 cups mixed vegetables

PM SNACK (OPTIONAL)

Men

1 cup blackberries or other berries
in season

Women

1 cup blackberries or other berries
in season

BREAKFAST

TUESDAY

Men

4 scrambled egg whites or 1 serving
Turkey Sausage Patties (page 192)
1 serving Fruit Shake (page 220) (or ½ cup
mixed berries)

Women

3 scrambled egg whites or ½ serving
Turkey Sausage Patties (page 192)
1 serving Fruit Shake (page 220)
(or ½ cup mixed berries)

MIDMORNING SNACK

Men

4 oz. baked turkey breast

1 to 2 cups greens (any type) with
    Cucumber Vinaigrette (page 213)

Women

3 oz. baked turkey breast

1 to 2 cups greens (any type) with
    Cucumber Vinaigrette (page 213)

LUNCH

Men

1 serving Steeped Chicken (page 199)
    or 4 oz. baked chicken breast

1 cup rice

1 to 2 cups mixed vegetables

Women

½ serving Steeped Chicken (page 199)
    or 2 oz. baked chicken breast

½ cup rice

1 to 2 cups mixed vegetables

MIDAFTERNOON SNACK

Men

4 oz. fresh tuna or no-sodium-added
    canned tuna

1 to 2 cups greens (any type) with
    Cucumber Vinaigrette (page 213)

Women

3 oz. fresh tuna or no-sodium-added
    canned tuna

1 to 2 cups greens (any type) with
    Cucumber Vinaigrette (page 213)

DINNER

Men

1 serving Chicken and Asparagus
    Stir-Fry (page 196) or 4 oz. baked
    chicken breast with 1 to 2 cups mixed
    vegetables

1 cup brown rice

Women

½ serving Chicken and Asparagus
    Stir-Fry (page 196) or 2 oz. baked
    chicken breast with 1 to 2 cups mixed
    vegetables

½ cup brown rice

PM SNACK (OPTIONAL)

Men

1 grapefruit

Women

1 grapefruit

TUESDAY

BREAKFAST

Men

1 serving Egg White Meringue Cookies
(page 221, made with 4 egg whites)
or 1 serving Turkey Sausage Patties
(page 192)

½ cup sliced strawberries

Women

1 serving Egg White Meringue Cookies
(page 221, made with 3 egg whites)
or ½ serving Turkey Sausage Patties
(page 192)

½ cup sliced strawberries

MIDMORNING SNACK

Men

4 oz. baked turkey breast (plain or with
Indian Marinade—page 184)

1 to 2 cups greens (any type) with
Cucumber Vinaigrette (page 213)

Women

3 oz. baked turkey breast (plain or with
Indian Marinade—page 184)

1 to 2 cups greens (any type) with
Cucumber Vinaigrette (page 213)

LUNCH

Men

4 oz. baked chicken breast

1 to 2 cups mixed vegetables

1 cup Rice Pudding for dessert
(page 222)

Women

2 oz. baked chicken breast

1 to 2 cups mixed vegetables

½ cup Rice Pudding for dessert
(page 222)

MIDAFTERNOON SNACK

Men

4 oz. Grilled Tuna Steak (page 188)
or no-sodium-added canned tuna

1 to 2 cups greens (any type) with
Cucumber Vinaigrette (page 213)

Women

3 oz. Grilled Tuna Steak (page 188)
or no-sodium-added canned tuna

1 to 2 cups greens (any type) with
Cucumber Vinaigrette (page 213)

DINNER

Men	Women
4 oz. Orange and Garlic Chicken (page 193) or 4 oz. baked chicken breast	2 oz. Orange and Garlic Chicken (page 193) or 2 oz. baked chicken breast
1 cup brown rice	½ cup brown rice
1 to 2 cups Summer Squash Medley (page 208) or 1 to 2 cups mixed vegetables	1 to 2 cups Summer Squash Medley (page 208) or 1 to 2 cups mixed vegetables

WEDNESDAY

PM SNACK (OPTIONAL)

Men	Women
1 Broiled Cinnamon Grapefruit (page 221)	1 Broiled Cinnamon Grapefruit (page 221)

BREAKFAST

Men	Women
1 serving Turkey Sausage Patties (page 192) or 4 oz. turkey breast	½ serving Turkey Sausage Patties (page 192) or 2 oz. turkey breast
½ grapefruit (or ½ cup mixed berries)	½ grapefruit (or ½ cup mixed berries)

MIDMORNING SNACK

Men	Women
4 oz. baked turkey breast (baked plain or in Cuban Lime Marinade—page 184)	3 oz. baked turkey breast (baked plain or in Cuban Lime Marinade—page 184)
1 to 2 cups greens (any type) with Cucumber Vinaigrette (page 213)	1 to 2 cups greens (any type) with Cucumber Vinaigrette (page 213)

THURSDAY

LUNCH

Men	Women
4 oz. baked chicken breast	2 oz. baked chicken breast
1 cup Spanish Rice (page 211)	½ cup Spanish Rice (page 211)
1 to 2 cups mixed vegetables	1 to 2 cups mixed vegetables

MIDAFTERNOON SNACK

Men

4 oz. fresh tuna or no-sodium-added
   canned tuna

1 to 2 cups greens (any type) with
   Cucumber Vinaigrette (page 213)

Women

3 oz. fresh tuna or no-sodium-added
   canned tuna

1 to 2 cups greens (any type) with
   Cucumber Vinaigrette (page 213)

DINNER

Men

1 serving Poached Chicken (page 197) or
   4 oz. baked chicken breast

1 cup brown rice

1 to 2 cups Ratatouille (page 206) or 1 to
   2 cups mixed vegetables

Women

½ serving Poached Chicken (page 197) or
   2 oz. baked chicken breast

½ cup brown rice

1 to 2 cups Ratatouille (page 206) or 1 to
   2 cups mixed vegetables

PM SNACK (OPTIONAL)

Men

1 grapefruit or 1 cup mixed berries

Women

1 grapefruit or 1 cup mixed berries

BREAKFAST

Men

4 scrambled egg whites or 1 serving
   Turkey Sausage Patties (page 192)

½ grapefruit (or ½ cup mixed berries)

Women

3 scrambled egg whites or ½ serving
   Turkey Sausage Patties (page 192)

½ grapefruit (or ½ cup mixed berries)

MIDMORNING SNACK

Men

4 oz. baked turkey breast

1 to 2 cups greens (any type) with
   Cucumber Vinaigrette (page 213)

Women

3 oz. baked turkey breast

1 to 2 cups greens (any type) with
   Cucumber Vinaigrette (page 213)

LUNCH

Men

4 oz. baked chicken breast

1 cup Wild Mushroom and Tomato Rice
  (page 212)

1 cup mixed greens (any type)

Women

2 oz. baked chicken breast

½ cup Wild Mushroom and Tomato Rice
  (page 212)

1 cup mixed greens (any type)

MIDAFTERNOON SNACK

Men

4 oz. Grilled Tuna Steak (page 188)
  or no-sodium-added canned tuna

1 to 2 cups Cucumber Salad (page 215)

Women

3 oz. Grilled Tuna Steak (page 188)
  or no-sodium-added canned tuna

1 to 2 cups Cucumber Salad (page 215)

DINNER

Men

4 oz. Orange and Garlic Chicken
  (page 193) or 4 oz. baked chicken
  breast

1 cup brown rice

1 to 2 cups Spicy Asparagus (page 208) or
  1 to 2 cups mixed vegetables

Women

2 oz. Orange and Garlic Chicken
  (page 193) or 2 oz. baked chicken
  breast

½ cup brown rice

1 to 2 cups Spicy Asparagus (page 208) or
  1 to 2 cups mixed vegetables

PM SNACK (OPTIONAL)

Men

1 cup Strawberry Delight (page 219)

Women

1 cup Strawberry Delight (page 219)

FRIDAY

Body Type D (Endo-Ecto)

With Body Type D—your shape may resemble an oval, with a fuller chest, less defined waist, and narrow shoulders and legs—two factors work together to cause your body to gain weight: a sluggish metabolism and a lack of lean muscle. The fact that your body has less lean muscle means it can't burn as many calories, and that further slows down your metabolic rate. This plan, however, will cause your body to gain and retain lean muscle (provided you are exercising with both cardiovascular and weight training).

Dieting is a serious problem for Body Type D's, because one of the downsides of dieting is that you start restricting calories; as a consequence, your body starts losing muscle tissue. The more muscle it loses, the less able your body is to burn up calories, and the more sluggish your metabolism becomes. In many ways, for a Type D, the less you eat, the more you gain.

The types and quantities of carbohydrates and proteins you eat will have a dramatic effect on the speed of your metabolism and its ability to maintain muscle—and, in turn, the rate at which your body loses or gains weight. Even more than other body types, you must be careful about the kind of carbohydrates you eat. Processed and simple carbohydrates dismantle easily into sugar, which means they hit your bloodstream rapidly. This provokes a spike in insulin levels, which leads to greater fat storage. You will need to eat more complex carbs because they are converted less quickly to sugar and will not slow down your metabolism.

You'll also need to carefully balance the ratio of carbohydrates to certain proteins. This is easy, though, since the six-day plan does it for you—no guesswork, no cumbersome calculations. While some body types don't have as much of a problem with relatively high levels of carbs and fruits in combination with smaller amounts of protein, this is not true of Body Type D. In your body, eating too many of the wrong types of carbs or eating carbohydrates alone, without protein or another type of food to slow down their conversion to sugar, can essentially bring your metabolism to a halt and make it very difficult to lose any weight.

Because your body is quite sensitive to insulin elevations, you'll do best by eating slightly smaller quantities of carbohydrates relative to protein. To really get your body shedding pounds and inches this week, you'll need to emphasize the complex carbohydrates as your primary source of these energy foods. You can also eat nearly all the green vegetables you desire because they have very few calories and almost no effect on metabolism.

Eating lean, high-quality protein has special benefits for Body Type D's and is more important for you than it is for nearly any of the other body types. Note that poultry, fish, and red meat are permissible in your diet. Red meat, in particular, has an important advantage for you because beef contains iron, vitamin B_{12}, and certain amino acids that will help enhance lean muscle on your body. Another top-drawer nutrient in red meat is creatine, which is involved in building body-defining muscle. Creatine is also responsible for boosting the pace of energy production in your cells, so to some degree it helps you push harder and longer in workouts. Because one of the biggest problems for a Body Type D is insufficient muscle, any nutrient that will assist in toning and firming lean muscle (in partnership with exercise) will accelerate your metabolism, burn more calories, and help you lose weight.

Caution: When I say you can eat red meat, I'm not talking about sausage and cheeseburgers! You'll need to choose the very leanest cuts of meat because fat will slow your metabolism. Also bear in mind that red meat can increase cholesterol levels, so if you suffer from that health condition, please choose other proteins such as poultry or fish.

Body Type D Makeover: Permissible Foods List

Proteins			Carbohydrates		Vegetables	Greens
Poultry	**Lean Beef**	**Fish**	**Starches**	**Fruits**		
Egg whites	Arm chuck	Bass	Brown rice	Blackberries	Alfalfa sprouts	Arugula
Chicken	pot roast	Catfish	Long-grain	Blueberries	Asparagus	Beet greens
breast, skin	Bottom round	Cod	rice	Boysenberries	Broccoli	Collard
removed	Eye of round	Flounder	Wild rice	Grapefruit	Brussels sprouts	greens
Chicken	Round tip	Grouper		Raspberries	Cabbage	Dandelion
breast,	(sirloin	Haddock		Strawberries	Cauliflower	greens
ground	tip)	Halibut			Celery	Endive
Turkey breast,	Tenderloin	Monkfish			Cucumber	Kale
skin	Top Loin	Orange			Eggplant	Lettuce, all
removed	(strip loin)	roughy			Garlic	varieties

Proteins				Vegetables	Greens
Poultry	**Lean Beef**	**Fish**			
Turkey breast,	Top round	Perch		Green beans	Mustard
ground	Top sirloin	Pollack		Mushrooms	greens
		Red snapper		Okra	Parsley
		Salmon		Onions	Spinach
		Shark		Pea pods	Swiss chard
		Sole		Peppers, all	Turnip greens
		Swordfish		varieties	Watercress
		Tilapia		Scallions	
		Trout		Summer	
		Tuna		squash, all	
		(fresh or		varieties	
		no-sodium-		Zucchini	
		added			
		canned)			
		Whitefish			

The *6-Day Body Makeover* Eating Plan for Body Type D

The Body Type D Eating Plan specifies exactly what you should eat (and in what quantities) for the next six days. I've provided a template for you, to show you the basics of a typical day on the Body Type D Eating Plan. In the section that follows this template, you'll find a day-by-day eating plan for Body Type D. This plan tells you exactly what to eat on each of the six days and is designed to remove all the guesswork from your meal planning. The recipes suggested here can be found in appendix A. If you are a Body Type D, you should commit to a weight-training program like the one described in chapter 8 for building muscle, since you have very little muscle tissue on your frame.

Very important:

- Do not deviate from the permissible foods that were listed previously or are listed in your menus.

- Follow your eating plan exactly with regard to the food suggestions. *Make no substitutions* for the suggested food unless you're substituting lean poultry for fish.

- If you don't like the suggested recipe or would prefer a different method of preparation, check appendix A for an alternative recipe that suits your body type.

- Pay strict attention to portion sizes.

- Do not use oil, mayonnaise, salad dressings (except those in appendix A), butter, margarine, vegetable oil spray, or any other added oils or fats.

- Never skip any meals, except for the optional PM snack.

- Drink 100 ounces (approximately twelve 8-ounce glasses) of water daily.

A Typical Day — Eating Plan Template for Body Type D

BREAKFAST

Men: 4 oz. lean beef and 3 to 4 scrambled egg whites (or 3 to 4 oz. turkey sausage)

Women: 3 oz. lean beef and 2 to 3 scrambled egg whites (or 2 to 3 oz. turkey sausage)

MIDMORNING SNACK

Men: 4 oz. lean beef (or chicken breast) and 1 cup greens (any type)

Women: 3 oz. lean beef (or chicken breast) and 1 cup greens (any type)

LUNCH

Men: 5 oz. chicken breast, 1 cup rice, and 1 cup mixed vegetables

Women: 2 to 3 oz. chicken breast, ½ cup rice, and 1 cup mixed vegetables

MIDAFTERNOON SNACK

Men: 4 oz. chicken breast and 1 cup mixed greens (any type)

Women: 3 oz. chicken breast and 1 cup mixed greens (any type)

DINNER

Men: 5 oz. chicken breast, 1 cup rice, and 1 cup mixed vegetables

Women: 2 to 3 oz. chicken breast, ½ cup rice, and 1 cup mixed vegetables

Men: 2 to 3 oz. fresh tuna or no-sodium-added canned tuna and 1 cup mixed greens (any type)

Women: 1 to 2 oz. fresh tuna or no-sodium-added canned tuna and 1 cup mixed greens (any type)

Day-by-Day Eating Plan for Body Type D (with Recipes)

BREAKFAST

Men	Women
4 oz. lean beef	3 oz. lean beef
3 to 4 scrambled egg whites or 1 serving Turkey Sausage Patties (page 192)	2 to 3 scrambled egg whites or ½ serving Turkey Sausage Patties (page 192)

MIDMORNING SNACK

Men	Women
4 oz. lean beef or chicken breast	3 oz. lean beef or chicken breast
1 cup greens (any type) with Cucumber Vinaigrette (page 213)	1 cup greens (any type) with Cucumber Vinaigrette (page 213)

LUNCH

Men	Women
2 Stuffed Peppers (page 195) or 5 oz. chicken breast with 1 cup rice and 1 cup mixed vegetables	1 Stuffed Pepper (page 195) or 2 to 3 oz. chicken breast with ½ cup rice and 1 cup mixed vegetables

MIDAFTERNOON SNACK

Men	Women
4 oz. baked chicken breast	3 oz. baked chicken breast
1 cup Gazpacho (page 207) or 1 cup mixed greens (any type)	1 cup Gazpacho (page 207) or 1 cup mixed greens (any type)

SUNDAY

DINNER

Men

1 serving Spicy Chicken (page 198) or
   5 oz. baked chicken breast

1 cup rice

1 cup Green Bean Salad (page 216) or
   1 cup mixed vegetables

Women

½ serving Spicy Chicken (page 198) or
   2 to 3 oz. baked chicken breast

½ cup rice

1 cup Green Bean Salad (page 216) or
   1 cup mixed vegetables

PM SNACK (OPTIONAL)

Men

2 to 3 oz. fresh tuna or no-sodium-added
   canned tuna

1 cup Cucumber Salad (page 215) or
   1 cup mixed greens (any type)

Women

1 to 2 oz. fresh tuna or no-sodium-added
   canned tuna

1 cup Cucumber Salad (page 215) or
   1 cup mixed greens (any type)

BREAKFAST

Men

4 oz. lean beef

1 serving Egg White Meringue Cookies
   (page 221, made with 4 egg whites) or
   4 scrambled egg whites

Women

3 oz. lean beef

1 serving Egg White Meringue Cookies
   (page 221, made with 3 egg whites) or
   2 to 3 scrambled egg whites

MIDMORNING SNACK

Men

4 oz. lean beef (or chicken breast)

1 cup greens (any type) with Cucumber
   Vinaigrette (page 213)

Women

3 oz. lean beef (or chicken breast)

1 cup greens (any type) with Cucumber
   Vinaigrette (page 213)

LUNCH

Men

5 oz. chicken breast

1 cup Spanish Rice (page 211)

1 cup mixed vegetables

Women

2 to 3 oz. chicken breast

½ cup Spanish Rice (page 211)

1 cup mixed vegetables

MIDAFTERNOON SNACK

Men

4 oz. baked chicken breast

1 cup mixed greens (any type)

Women

3 oz. baked chicken breast

1 cup mixed greens (any type)

DINNER

Men

1 serving Lemon Oregano Chicken
(page 197) or 5 oz. baked chicken
breast

1 cup rice

1 cup Green Bean Salad (page 216) or
1 cup mixed vegetables

Women

½ serving Lemon Oregano Chicken
(page 197) or 2 to 3 oz. baked chicken
breast

½ cup rice

1 cup Green Bean Salad (page 216) or
1 cup mixed vegetables

PM SNACK (OPTIONAL)

Men

2 to 3 oz. fresh tuna or no-sodium-added
canned tuna

1 cup mixed greens (any type)

Women

1 to 2 oz. fresh tuna or no-sodium-added
canned tuna

1 cup mixed greens (any type)

BREAKFAST

TUESDAY

Men

4 oz. lean beef

3 to 4 scrambled egg whites or 1 serving
Turkey Sausage Patties (page 192)

Women

3 oz. lean beef

2 to 3 scrambled egg whites or ½ serving
Turkey Sausage Patties (page 192)

MIDMORNING SNACK

Men

4 oz. lean beef (or chicken breast)

1 cup Summer Squash Medley (page 208)
or 1 cup greens (any type)

Women

3 oz. lean beef (or chicken breast)

1 cup Summer Squash Medley (page 208)
or 1 cup greens (any type)

Customized Eating Plans   91

LUNCH

Men	Women
1 serving Spicy Chicken (page 198) or 5 oz. chicken breast	½ serving Spicy Chicken (page 198) or 2 to 3 oz. chicken breast
1 cup rice	½ cup rice
1 cup mixed vegetables	1 cup mixed vegetables

MIDAFTERNOON SNACK

Men	Women
4 oz. baked chicken breast	3 oz. baked chicken breast
1 cup Colorful Cabbage Slaw (page 213) or 1 cup mixed greens (any type)	1 cup Colorful Cabbage Slaw (page 213) or 1 cup mixed greens (any type)

DINNER

Men	Women
5 oz. baked chicken breast	2 to 3 oz. chicken breast
1 cup rice	½ cup rice
1 cup Ratatouille (page 206) or 1 cup mixed vegetables	1 cup Ratatouille (page 206) or 1 cup mixed vegetables

PM SNACK (OPTIONAL)

Men	Women
2 to 3 oz. Grilled Tuna Steak (page 188) or no-sodium-added canned tuna	1 to 2 oz. Grilled Tuna Steak (page 188) or no-sodium-added canned tuna
1 cup mixed greens (any type)	1 cup mixed greens (any type)

BREAKFAST

Men	Women
4 oz. lean beef	3 oz. lean beef
3 to 4 scrambled egg whites or 1 serving Turkey Sausage Patties (page 192)	2 to 3 scrambled egg whites or ½ serving Turkey Sausage Patties (page 192)

TUESDAY

WEDNESDAY

MIDMORNING SNACK

Men

4 oz. lean beef (or chicken breast)

1 cup Gazpacho (page 207) or 1 cup
mixed greens (any type)

Women

3 oz. lean beef (or chicken breast)

1 cup Gazpacho (page 207) or 1 cup
mixed greens (any type)

LUNCH

Men

5 oz. chicken breast

1 cup Wild Mushroom and Tomato Rice
(page 212)

Women

2 to 3 oz. chicken breast

½ cup Wild Mushroom and Tomato Rice
(page 212)

MIDAFTERNOON SNACK

Men

4 oz. baked chicken breast

1 cup Mexican Salad (page 214) or 1 cup
mixed greens (any type)

Women

3 oz. baked chicken breast

1 cup Mexican Salad (page 214) or 1 cup
mixed greens (any type)

DINNER

Men

1 serving Jamaican Chicken (page 200) or
5 oz. baked chicken breast

1 cup rice

1 cup Grilled Vegetables (page 205) or
1 cup mixed vegetables

Women

½ serving Jamaican Chicken (page 200)
or 2 to 3 oz. baked chicken breast

½ cup rice

1 cup Grilled Vegetables (page 205) or
1 cup mixed vegetables

PM SNACK (OPTIONAL)

Men

2 to 3 oz. fresh tuna or no-sodium-added
canned tuna

1 cup Cucumber Salad (page 215) or
1 cup mixed greens (any type)

Women

1 to 2 oz. fresh tuna or no-sodium-added
canned tuna

1 cup Cucumber Salad (page 215) or
1 cup mixed greens (any type)

BREAKFAST

Men

4 oz. lean beef

1 serving Egg White Meringue Cookies
    (page 221, made with 4 egg whites) or
    4 scrambled egg whites

Women

3 oz. lean beef

1 serving Egg White Meringue Cookies
    (page 221, made with 3 egg whites) or
    2 to 3 scrambled egg whites

MIDMORNING SNACK

Men

4 oz. lean beef or chicken breast

1 cup Spicy Asparagus (page 208) or
    1 cup mixed greens (any type)

Women

3 oz. lean beef (or chicken breast)

1 cup Spicy Asparagus (page 208) or
    1 cup mixed greens (any type)

LUNCH

Men

2 Stuffed Peppers (page 195) or 5 oz.
    chicken breast with 1 cup rice and
    1 cup mixed vegetables

Women

1 Stuffed Pepper (page 195) or 2 to 3 oz.
    chicken breast with ½ cup rice and
    1 cup mixed vegetables

MIDAFTERNOON SNACK

Men

4 oz. baked chicken breast (plain or with
    Cuban Lime Marinade—page 184)

1 cup mixed greens (any type)

Women

3 oz. baked chicken breast (plain or with
    Cuban Lime Marinade—page 184)

1 cup mixed greens (any type)

DINNER

Men

1 serving Orange and Garlic Chicken
    (page 193) or 5 oz. baked chicken
    breast with 1 cup rice and 1 cup
    Cucumber Salad (page 215) or 1 cup
    mixed vegetables

Women

½ serving Orange and Garlic Chicken
    (page 193) or 2 to 3 oz. baked chicken
    breast with ½ cup rice and 1 cup
    Cucumber Salad (page 215) or 1 cup
    mixed vegetables

THURSDAY

PM SNACK (OPTIONAL)

Men	*Women*
2 to 3 oz. fresh tuna or no-sodium-added canned tuna	1 to 2 oz. fresh tuna or no-sodium-added canned tuna
1 cup mixed greens (any type) with Cucumber Vinaigrette (page 213)	1 cup mixed greens (any type) with Cucumber Vinaigrette (page 213)

BREAKFAST

Men	*Women*
4 oz. lean beef	3 oz. lean beef
3 to 4 scrambled egg whites or 1 serving Turkey Sausage Patties (page 192)	2 to 3 scrambled egg whites or ½ serving Turkey Sausage Patties (page 192)

MIDMORNING SNACK

Men	*Women*
4 oz. lean beef (or chicken breast)	3 oz. lean beef (or chicken breast)
1 cup Mexican Salad (page 214) or 1 cup mixed greens (any type)	1 cup Mexican Salad (page 214) or 1 cup mixed greens (any type)

LUNCH

Men	*Women*
5 oz. chicken breast	2 to 3 oz. chicken breast
1 cup mixed vegetables	1 cup mixed vegetables
1 cup Rice Pudding for dessert (page 222)	½ cup Rice Pudding for dessert (page 222)

MIDAFTERNOON SNACK

Men	*Women*
1 serving Steeped Chicken (page 199) or 4 oz. baked chicken breast	½ serving Steeped Chicken (page 199) or 3 oz. baked chicken breast
1 cup zucchini or 1 cup mixed greens (any type)	1 cup zucchini or 1 cup mixed greens (any type)

FRIDAY

Men

5 oz. baked chicken breast (plain or with Indian Marinade—page 184)

1 cup rice

1 cup Colorful Cabbage Slaw (page 213) or 1 cup mixed vegetables

Women

2 to 3 oz. baked chicken breast (plain or with Indian Marinade—page 184)

½ cup rice

1 cup Colorful Cabbage Slaw (page 213) or 1 cup mixed vegetables

PM SNACK (OPTIONAL)

Men

2 to 3 oz. fresh tuna or no-sodium-added canned tuna

1 cup Cucumber Salad (page 215) or 1 cup mixed greens (any type)

Women

1 to 2 oz. fresh tuna or no-sodium-added canned tuna

1 cup Cucumber Salad (page 215) or 1 cup mixed greens (any type)

Body Type E (Ecto-Endo)

The goal of your eating plan is to keep your metabolism moving fast enough to burn fat, while causing it to add and maintain the lean muscle that will give you a shapely, well-defined body so that you can burn even more fat. With a Body Type E, your physique may resemble a tube, with a skinny, bony frame underneath areas of body fat.

Because part of your body is endomorphic, eating too many of the wrong carbs, or eating carbs alone without protein, can essentially bring your metabolism to a halt. Therefore, you will eat more slow carbs and fewer fast carbs or simple sugars. The specific slow carbs on your eating plan are converted less quickly to sugar and therefore won't interfere with your metabolic rate.

Fortunately, though, your metabolism isn't as slow as some of the other body types. That means your eating plan includes slightly more carbohydrates than other meal plans. However, you must be vigilant about the types and quantities of carbohydrates you eat. In addition, stay away from sweet fruits such as cherries, oranges, or watermelon, since these will further slow down your somewhat sluggish metabolism.

Your meal plan also includes beans, a slow carb that contains more protein than most vegetables. Beans are a nutrient powerhouse packed with not only protein but also fiber, B-complex vitamins, and minerals. With the exception of soybeans, most beans are incomplete proteins, because they lack one or more essential amino acids. Nonetheless, they turn into complete proteins when combined in meals with grains (such as rice) and animal proteins, as your eating plan does. These foods supply the missing amino acids to complement the protein in beans.

For Body Type E, eating protein in sufficient amounts and eating it often are more important than for any of the other body types. The reason for this is that your body already has trouble maintaining muscle tissue, so a constant supply of protein is required to build and repair body tissues, as well as maintain strong muscles. The more muscle you can develop, the more resistant your body becomes to future weight gain. Your eating plan will ensure that you get enough of the right types of protein (and carbs) in just the right amounts and at the right times.

For animal protein, you have more selections than almost any of the other body types. While I encourage people with other body types to eat mostly fish and lean poultry,

I recommend that Body Type E's consume more red meat. Red meat is particularly advantageous because it supplies higher levels of creatine and amino acids—nutrients that are involved in enhancing lean, shapely muscle on your body. Your red meat choices, however, must be lean to minimize your fat intake.

As I have noted, one of the biggest challenges for you is insufficient muscle. Anything that will help you increase the size of your muscles will speed up your metabolism, burn more fat, give your body shape, and stimulate weight loss. Your eating plan is geared toward these goals. As a Body Type E, you should definitely commit to a weight-training program, like the one described in chapter 8, for building muscle, since you have very little muscle tissue on your frame.

Body Type E Makeover: Permissible Foods List

Proteins			Carbohydrates		Vegetables	Greens
Poultry	**Lean Beef**	**Fish**	**Starches**	**Fruits**		
Egg whites	Arm chuck	Bass	Brown rice	Blackberries	Alfalfa sprouts	Arugula
Chicken	pot roast	Catfish	Long-grain	Blueberries	Asparagus	Beet greens
breast, skin	Bottom round	Cod	rice	Boysenberries	Broccoli	Collard
removed	Eye of round	Flounder	Wild rice	Grapefruit	Brussels sprouts	greens
Chicken	Round tip	Grouper	Black beans	Raspberries	Cabbage	Dandelion
breast,	(sirloin tip)	Haddock	Broad beans	Strawberries	Cauliflower	greens
ground	Tenderloin	Halibut	(fava)		Celery	Endive
Turkey breast,	Top loin	Monkfish	Chickpeas		Cucumber	Kale
skin	(strip loin)	Orange	(garbanzo)		Eggplant	Lettuce, all
removed	Top round	roughy	Cranberry		Garlic	varieties
Turkey breast,	Top sirloin	Perch	beans		Green beans	Mustard
ground		Pollack	Great north-		Mushrooms	greens
		Red snapper	ern beans		Okra	Parsley
		Salmon	Kidney beans		Onions	Spinach
		Shark	Lima beans		Pea pods	Swiss chard
		Sole	Navy beans		Peppers, all	Turnip greens
		Swordfish	Pink beans		varieties	Watercress
		Tilapia	Pinto beans		Scallions	
		Trout	White beans			

Proteins			Vegetables	Greens
Poultry	**Lean Beef**	**Fish**		
		Tuna (fresh or no-sodium-added canned)	Summer squash, all varieties	
		Whitefish	Zucchini	

The *6-Day Body Makeover* Eating Plan for Body Type E

The Body Type E Eating Plan specifies exactly what you should eat (and in what quantities) for the next six days. I've provided a template for you, to show you the basics of a typical day on the Body Type E Eating Plan. In the section that follows this template, you'll find a day-by-day eating plan for Body Type E. This plan tells you exactly what to eat on each of the six days and is designed to remove all the guesswork from your meal planning. The recipes suggested here can be found in appendix A.

Very important:

- Do not deviate from the permissible foods that were listed previously or are listed in your menus.

- Follow your eating plan exactly with regard to the food suggestions. *Make no substitutions* for the suggested food unless you're substituting lean poultry for fish.

- If you don't like the suggested recipe or would prefer a different method of preparation, check appendix A for an alternative recipe that suits your body type.

- Pay strict attention to portion sizes.

- Do not use oil, mayonnaise, salad dressings (except those in appendix A), butter, margarine, vegetable oil spray, or any other added oils or fats.

- Never skip any meals, except for the optional PM snack.

- Drink 100 ounces (approximately twelve 8-ounce glasses) of water daily.

A Typical Day — Eating Plan Template for Body Type E

BREAKFAST

Men: 4 oz. lean beef and 4 to 5 scrambled egg whites (or 4 to 5 oz. turkey sausage)

Women: 3 oz. lean beef and 2 to 3 scrambled egg whites (or 2 to 3 oz. turkey sausage)

MIDMORNING SNACK

Men: 4 to 5 oz. lean beef (or chicken breast) and 1 to 2 cups mixed greens (any type)

Women: 3 oz. lean beef (or chicken breast) and 1 to 2 cups mixed greens (any type)

LUNCH

Men: 5 oz. chicken breast, ½ cup beans and ½ cup rice, and 1 to 2 cups mixed vegetables

Women: 2 to 3 oz. chicken breast, ¼ cup beans and ¼ cup rice, and 1 to 2 cups mixed vegetables

MIDAFTERNOON SNACK

Men: 4 oz. lean beef and 1 grapefruit (or 1 cup mixed berries)

Women: 3 oz. lean beef and 1 grapefruit (or 1 cup mixed berries)

DINNER

Men: 5 oz. chicken breast, ½ cup beans and ½ cup rice, and 1 to 2 cups mixed vegetables

Women: 2 to 3 oz. chicken breast, ¼ cup beans and ¼ cup rice, and 1 to 2 cups mixed vegetables

PM SNACK (OPTIONAL)

Men: 2 to 3 oz. chicken breast and ½ grapefruit (or ½ cup mixed berries)

Women: 1 to 2 oz. chicken breast and ½ grapefruit (or ½ cup mixed berries)

Day-by-Day Eating Plan for Body Type E

BREAKFAST

Men

4 oz. lean beef

4 to 5 scrambled egg whites or 1 serving
Turkey Sausage Patties (page 192)

Women

3 oz. lean beef

2 to 3 scrambled egg whites or ½ serving
Turkey Sausage Patties (page 192)

MIDMORNING SNACK

Men

4 to 5 oz. lean beef (or chicken breast)

1 to 2 cups Mexican Salad (page 214) or
1 to 2 cups mixed greens (any type)

Women

3 oz. lean beef (or chicken breast)

1 to 2 cups Mexican Salad (page 214) or
1 to 2 cups mixed greens (any type)

LUNCH

Men

1 serving Steeped Chicken (page 199) or
5 oz. baked chicken breast

½ cup beans and ½ cup rice

1 to 2 cups mixed vegetables

Women

½ serving Steeped Chicken (page 199) or
2 to 3 oz. baked chicken breast

¼ cup beans and ¼ cup rice

1 to 2 cups mixed vegetables

MIDAFTERNOON SNACK

Men

4 oz. lean beef

1 grapefruit (or 1 cup mixed berries)

Women

3 oz. lean beef

1 grapefruit (or 1 cup mixed berries)

DINNER

Men

1 serving Jamaican Chicken (page 200) or
5 oz. chicken breast

½ cup beans and ½ cup rice

1 to 2 cups Grilled Vegetables (page 205)

Women

½ serving Jamaican Chicken (page 200)
or 2 to 3 oz. chicken breast

¼ cup beans and ¼ cup rice

1 to 2 cups Grilled Vegetables (page 205)

PM SNACK (OPTIONAL)

Men

2 to 3 oz. chicken breast

½ grapefruit (or ½ cup mixed berries)

Women

1 to 2 oz. chicken breast

½ grapefruit (or ½ cup mixed berries)

BREAKFAST

Men

4 oz. lean beef

4 to 5 scrambled egg whites or 1 serving
   Turkey Sausage Patties (page 192)

Women

3 oz. lean beef

2 to 3 scrambled egg whites or ½ serving
   Turkey Sausage Patties (page 192)

MIDMORNING SNACK

Men

4 to 5 oz. lean beef (or chicken breast)

1 to 2 cups Green Bean Salad (page 216)
   or 1 to 2 cups greens (any type)

Women

3 oz. lean beef (or chicken breast)

1 to 2 cups Green Bean Salad (page 216)
   or 1 to 2 cups greens (any type)

LUNCH

Men

1 serving Five-Alarm Chili (page 201) or
   5 oz. chicken breast with ½ cup beans
   and ½ cup rice

1 to 2 cups mixed vegetables

Women

½ serving Five-Alarm Chili (page 201) or
   2 to 3 oz. chicken breast with ¼ cup
   beans and ¼ cup rice

1 to 2 cups mixed vegetables

MIDAFTERNOON SNACK

Men

4 oz. lean beef

1 cup Strawberry Delight (page 219)

Women

3 oz. lean beef

1 cup Strawberry Delight (page 219)

DINNER

Men

5 oz. chicken breast

½ cup beans and ½ cup rice

1 to 2 cups Colorful Cabbage Slaw
   (page 213)

Women

2 to 3 oz. chicken breast

¼ cup beans and ¼ cup rice

1 to 2 cups Colorful Cabbage Slaw
   (page 213)

PM SNACK (OPTIONAL)

Men

2 to 3 oz. chicken breast

½ grapefruit

Women

1 to 2 oz. chicken breast

½ grapefruit

BREAKFAST

Men

4 oz. lean beef

1 serving Egg White Meringue Cookies
   (page 221, made with 4 egg whites)
   or 1 serving Turkey Sausage Patties
   (page 192)

Women

3 oz. lean beef

1 serving Egg White Meringue Cookies
   (page 221, made with 3 egg whites)
   or ½ serving Turkey Sausage Patties
   (page 192)

MIDMORNING SNACK

Men

4 to 5 oz. lean beef or chicken breast

1 to 2 cups Cucumber Salad (page 215) or
   1 to 2 cups mixed greens (any type)

Women

3 oz. lean beef or chicken breast

1 to 2 cups Cucumber Salad (page 215)
   or 1 to 2 cups mixed greens (any type)

LUNCH

Men

1 serving Poached Chicken (page 197)
   or 5 oz. chicken breast

½ cup beans and ½ cup rice

1 to 2 cups mixed vegetables

Women

½ serving Poached Chicken (page 197)
   or 2 to 3 oz. chicken breast

¼ cup beans and ¼ cup rice

1 to 2 cups mixed vegetables

MIDAFTERNOON SNACK

Men

4 oz. lean beef

1 Broiled Cinnamon Grapefruit
   (page 221)

Women

3 oz. lean beef

1 Broiled Cinnamon Grapefruit
   (page 221)

DINNER

TUESDAY

Men	Women
1 serving Classic Meat Loaf prepared with ground chicken (page 202) or 5 oz. chicken breast	½ serving Classic Meat Loaf prepared with ground chicken (page 202) or 2 to 3 oz. chicken breast
1 cup beans	½ cup beans
1 to 2 cups Grilled Vegetables (page 205)	1 to 2 cups Grilled Vegetables (page 205)

PM SNACK (OPTIONAL)

Men	Women
2 to 3 oz. chicken breast	1 to 2 oz. chicken breast
½ cup mixed berries	½ cup mixed berries

BREAKFAST

WEDNESDAY

Men	Women
4 oz. lean beef	3 oz. lean beef
4 to 5 scrambled egg whites or 1 serving Turkey Sausage Patties (page 192)	2 to 3 scrambled egg whites or ½ serving Turkey Sausage Patties (page 192)

MIDMORNING SNACK

Men	Women
4 to 5 oz. lean beef or chicken breast	3 oz. lean beef or chicken breast
1 to 2 cups Ratatouille (page 206) or 1 to 2 cups mixed greens (any type)	1 to 2 cups Ratatouille (page 206) or 1 to 2 cups mixed greens (any type)

LUNCH

Men	Women
5 oz. chicken breast	2 to 3 oz. chicken breast
½ cup beans and ½ cup rice	¼ cup beans and ¼ cup rice
1 to 2 cups mixed vegetables	1 to 2 cups mixed vegetables

MIDAFTERNOON SNACK

Men

4 oz. lean beef

1 cup blueberries or other berries
  in season

Women

3 oz. lean beef

1 cup blueberries or other berries
  in season

DINNER

Men

5 oz. chicken breast prepared with Cuban
  Lime Marinade (page 184)

½ cup beans and ½ cup rice

1 to 2 cups mixed greens (any type) with
  Cucumber Vinaigrette (page 213)

Women

2 to 3 oz. chicken breast prepared with
  Cuban Lime Marinade (page 184)

¼ cup beans and ¼ cup rice

1 to 2 cups mixed greens (any type) with
  Cucumber Vinaigrette (page 213)

PM SNACK (OPTIONAL)

Men

2 to 3 oz. chicken breast

½ Broiled Cinnamon Grapefruit
  (page 221)

Women

1 to 2 oz. chicken breast

½ Broiled Cinnamon Grapefruit
  (page 221)

BREAKFAST

Men

4 oz. lean beef

4 to 5 scrambled egg whites or 1 serving
  Turkey Sausage Patties (page 192)

Women

3 oz. lean beef

2 to 3 scrambled egg whites or ½ serving
  Turkey Sausage Patties (page 192)

MIDMORNING SNACK

Men

4 to 5 oz. lean beef or chicken breast

1 to 2 cups mixed greens (any type) with
  Cucumber Vinaigrette (page 213)

Women

3 oz. lean beef or chicken breast

1 to 2 cups mixed greens (any type) with
  Cucumber Vinaigrette (page 213)

LUNCH

Men

1 serving Spicy Chicken (page 198) or
    5 oz. chicken breast
½ cup beans and ½ cup rice
1 to 2 cups Mexican Salad (page 214) or
    1 to 2 cups mixed vegetables

Women

½ serving Spicy Chicken (page 198) or
    2 to 3 oz. chicken breast
¼ cup beans and ¼ cup rice
1 to 2 cups Mexican Salad (page 214) or
    1 to 2 cups mixed vegetables

MIDAFTERNOON SNACK

Men

4 oz. lean beef
1 cup Fruit Shake (page 220)

Women

3 oz. lean beef
1 cup Fruit Shake (page 220)

DINNER

Men

1 serving Chicken and Asparagus Stir-Fry
    (page 196) or 5 oz. chicken breast
½ cup beans and ½ cup rice
1 cup mixed greens (any type)

Women

½ serving Chicken and Asparagus Stir-Fry
    (page 196) or 2 to 3 oz. chicken breast
¼ cup beans and ¼ cup rice
1 cup mixed greens (any type)

PM SNACK (OPTIONAL)

Men

2 to 3 oz. chicken breast
½ grapefruit

Women

1 to 2 oz. chicken breast
½ grapefruit

BREAKFAST

Men

4 oz. lean beef
1 serving Egg White Meringue Cookies
    (page 221, made with 4 egg whites)
    or 1 serving Turkey Sausage Patties
    (page 192)

Women

3 oz. lean beef
1 serving Egg White Meringue Cookies
    (page 221, made with 3 egg whites)
    or ½ serving Turkey Sausage Patties
    (page 192)

THURSDAY

FRIDAY

MIDMORNING SNACK

Men

4 to 5 oz. lean beef or chicken breast

1 to 2 cups Gazpacho (page 207) or 1 to
   2 cups mixed greens (any type)

Women

3 oz. lean beef or chicken breast

1 to 2 cups Gazpacho (page 207) or 1 to
   2 cups mixed greens (any type)

LUNCH

Men

1 serving Poached Chicken (page 197) or
   5 oz. chicken breast

½ cup beans and ½ cup rice

1 to 2 cups mixed vegetables

Women

½ serving Poached Chicken (page 197) or
   2 to 3 oz. chicken breast

¼ cup beans and ¼ cup rice

1 to 2 cups mixed vegetables

MIDAFTERNOON SNACK

Men

4 oz. lean beef

1 cup Strawberry Delight (page 219)

Women

3 oz. lean beef

1 cup Strawberry Delight (page 219)

DINNER

Men

1 serving Jamaican Chicken (page 200)
   or 5 oz. chicken breast

½ cup beans and ½ cup rice

1 to 2 cups Summer Squash Medley
   (page 208)

Women

½ serving Jamaican Chicken (page 200)
   or 2 to 3 oz. chicken breast

¼ cup beans and ¼ cup rice

1 to 2 cups Summer Squash Medley
   (page 208)

PM SNACK (OPTIONAL)

Men

2 to 3 oz. chicken breast

½ grapefruit

Women

1 to 2 oz. chicken breast

½ grapefruit

Using Nutritional Supplements

Although you'll probably be eating more healthfully than you ever have before, it always makes sense to take a high-quality multivitamin/mineral supplement to cover all your nutritional bases. That way, your body has all the nutrients it needs to stay strong, healthy, and energized, so that you can maximize your fat loss. Exercising also increases the body's demand for additional nutrients, which can be supplied through supplements.

I recommend that you take a high-quality calcium supplement as well, especially if you're a woman. The best choice is one formulated with calcium citrate (because it is better absorbed) and with vitamin D, manganese, and boron—three nutrients that assist your body in utilizing calcium. In addition, always take your calcium supplement with meals for better absorption. Check with your physician for the recommended dosage, based on your age and sex.

There is now overwhelming scientific evidence that multivitamin/mineral pills, now taken by more than half of all Americans, may modify your risk of developing some of the most feared and fatal diseases now plaguing us—cardiovascular disease, cancer, Alzheimer's disease, and other chronic diseases. Simply popping your vitamin pill every day is one of the most positive—and easiest—health moves you can make.

Looking Toward Day 1

There you have it—exactly what you should eat for the next six days. Now that you have your eating plan in place, I want to give you some additional information that will help you maximize your results, no matter what your body type. One of the other components for success is planning for it—in other words, getting in gear mentally and motivationally. Keep turning the pages, and you'll learn more secrets that will keep you on track.

CHAPTER 5

Staying on Track: Simple Secrets That Make It Easy and Foolproof

L aunching into the *6-Day Body Makeover* isn't something you do without preparation and planning. It's absolutely essential that you prepare your mind for the work ahead, so that you can stay mentally relaxed, emotionally supple, and focused on achieving your goals. Equally important is learning how to control weaknesses that lead to overeating. That's where planning enters the picture. This involves acquiring all the food you need for the next six days, getting rid of what you don't need, and planning your meals day by day so that there is simply no way you can fail at this program. You'll also need to know your starting point, which is why you'll need to step on the scales and take some measurements (bet you thought you were going to escape that one!). That way, six days from now, you can be amazed by your progress when you zip up that dress or pair of pants you've been dying to squeeze into. Preparation and planning—nothing else matters if you want to be successful.

It's generally best to start the *6-Day Body Makeover* on a Sunday. Use Saturday to familiarize yourself with the program, psych yourself up, shop for groceries, and organize and prepare your food for the six days that follow, so you have everything ready. The other advantage of starting on a Sunday is that you will drop a clothing size by the weekend—and look and feel fabulous.

Think of the following secrets as the safety patrol of makeover control. They'll keep you on track, plus deliver weight-control benefits by getting you in the right frame of mind for the next six days. They'll help you think positively about the changes you're about to make and equip you for long-term lifestyle changes in order to keep you from gaining the weight back. These secrets will encourage you to work around obstacles such as impulse eating and to promote the substitution of new, healthier habits. While you might be tempted to skip over them at first, you'll quickly discover that they're really on your side and will make the next six days—and beyond—easy and foolproof.

Secret #1: Create a Success Scenario

Because attitudes can make or break your chances for success, the starting line for the *6-Day Body Makeover* is really in your head. So the day before you begin the makeover, whether it's Saturday or some other day of the week, get your head straight.

For starters, be realistic. Nothing can sabotage your makeover program faster than the impossible dream. As anyone who has ever tried to lose weight knows, overblown expectations lead to disappointment and failure. Yes, it is possible to lose 10 to 15 or more pounds in six days, if you are already quite heavy. Some people who have less to lose may shed 2 to 4 pounds in six days, and that's a great accomplishment, too. If you've never been able to lose weight before, and all of a sudden you drop 2 pounds, that means your metabolism is shifting out of neutral and getting in gear for greater losses. Each pound lost, whether it's 2 pounds, 10 pounds, or more, is a success.

Another part of being realistic is knowing where your body loses weight first and last. The first place weight goes on is usually the last place it comes off. So if you've put a lot of weight on your hips, that's probably the last area it will come off. As I like to repeat: Everyone is different. Every *body* is different. Be realistic about how your body burns off pounds.

In addition to harboring unrealistic expectations, you can sabotage yourself with a negative attitude, such as a lack of belief that you can really lose weight or drop a size over the next six days. If that's your mind-set, you're doomed before you begin.

My advice is this: Don't think *I can't*; think *I can* and *I will*! You will achieve what you believe. If you believe you can do it, you will. When I was making the transition from an obese kid to competitive bodybuilder (and developing the foundation for the techniques that would later become my makeover programs), I used to fantasize about how I wanted to look—chiseled abs, large biceps, muscular shoulders, the whole package. I wasn't just wishing I had an in-shape physique; I was very specific about what I wanted to accomplish.

I'd start by finding images of the body I wanted to have. I'd study those images in detail. Then I'd imagine the fat melting off my body and my individual muscles changing shape in very specific ways. This process of mental concentration—which I called "daydreaming"—helped me stay focused on my goal and eventually played a huge part in helping me get exactly the body I wanted for bodybuilding competitions. Then one day, I looked in the mirror, and there it was: I could see the physique I envisioned for myself begin to emerge. It was very exciting. When you see yourself change, it is a very empowering experience.

Without knowing it, I was utilizing a technique that is widely known today as visualization. While this may still seem like daydreaming, the fact of the matter is that visualization is now widely accepted in a variety of disciplines to help people achieve fantastic goals. Visualization is what helps Olympic athletes and professional ball players perform at their personal best. It is what has helped many cancer patients overcome life-threatening illness. And it is what will allow you to achieve just about any goal you set for yourself.

The conception of an event, or an end point, in your mind is the beginning of its existence, and without a clear image of what the outcome will be, the manifestation of that event is almost impossible. In other words, if you don't know what you want and don't believe you can get it, you can't. However, if you have a clear picture of what you want to accomplish and the solid belief that you can make it happen, then success is almost guaranteed. In fact, one of the greatest pieces of art was born out of an artist's vision that was widely doubted. The great Renaissance artist Michelangelo once salvaged a piece of marble that had been rejected by other sculptors because it was too long and narrow. Those sculptors asked him, "Of what value is that strange piece of marble? What will you ever be able to sculpt from it?"

What Michelangelo saw in that misshapen chunk of marble was to be one of the greatest masterpieces of all time. He put his vision to work, chiseling, carving, and refining. When he was finished, there stood the statue of David.

Maybe right now you think your body is like a misshapen block of marble. But trust me, if you use your mind to envision what you can be, you will begin to make the right choices, the healthy choices, to become what you see in your mind's eye. Your mind is a very powerful force that can help you achieve your inner vision of your desired outer appearance. The body you see yourself achieving, no matter how "misshapen" you feel you look now, is ultimately the body you want and will have.

Over the next six days (and beyond, if you have more weight to lose), I'd like you to use the following step-by-step visualization techniques to help strengthen your resolve and improve your chances of success.

Step 1: Be still. Find a quiet, comfortable space that is private, pleasant, and inspiring—even if it's simply a corner of your bedroom—with no time pressure or distracting noises. Take the phone off the hook; turn off the television. There's no place you have to be, no problems you have to solve now. Just sit or lie comfortably, and close your eyes.

Step 2: Learn to relax. The calmer you are, the more easily your body will lose weight, because stress increases levels of hormones that cause the body to produce fat. I have learned that visualization tends to calm the mind, defuse negative emotion, and cultivate more healthful mental states. The key is a simple technique called Abdominal Breathing. (You'll find more details on this in chapter 6, and you'll learn how it helps burn fat.) Take a deep breath through your nose, filling your lower abdomen. Your abdomen should rise as you inhale, not your chest. Then as you exhale through your mouth, your abdomen should fall. Air eases in and air eases out, with a slow current of respiration that is steady. This is the natural, proper way to breathe that we have forgotten as we got older. Watch a baby sometime, and you'll see that this is exactly how he or she breathes. Most adult breathing is shallow and not deep enough. Deep breathing, or Abdominal Breathing, is very important to true relaxation and to make the mind–body connection that is so important to the achievement of your goals. Breathe deeply like this, and progressively relax your body, beginning with your feet and working your way up to the top of your head.

Step 3: Visualize your dream body as you lie in a relaxed state. In your mind's eye, picture yourself wearing that new outfit that's one size smaller than you are now, or that "skinny dress" currently hanging unworn in your closet. If it helps you to better visualize, find a picture of yourself (if you have one) in that outfit or at that smaller size. A picture can help you keep your goal in sight. With as much detail as possible, think about how you will feel physically and emotionally when you are at that size or how you will look in those smaller, better-fitting clothes you'll be able to buy. See yourself being pampered by those sales folks selling you new, formfitting clothes. Picture yourself at the event in which you are wearing those clothes and how great you'll look in them. Dream away! Make this scene as vivid as possible, using as many of your senses as you can. Notice how you look, what you can hear, smell, feel, and taste. Notice your surroundings, whether there are other people there, and anything else that is a part of the success scenario. Notice how good it feels to be in those clothes. If your mind has a tendency to wander, try making a tape to listen to each time you do your visualization. Record your own voice, or someone else's voice, guiding the process: telling each part of your body to relax, and telling yourself to notice how you look and feel. The more vivid you can make the "new you" in your mind, the more successful you will be.

Step 4: Repeat what's affirming and positive. Accompany your visualization by what is known as a mantra, meaning a personal sound that is meaningful to you. For this exercise, create a weight-loss mantra. Tell yourself: *I'm going to lose weight and fit into a smaller size . . . I'm going to look fabulous in my outfit . . . People are going to enjoy seeing me succeed . . . I love my body, and I'll love it more when I lose those pounds.* Direct your thoughts and concentration to what is affirming, what is positive. Creating an unshakable positive attitude is critical to your achievement, and your affirmations, or mantra, will help you do it.

Step 5: Practice. Do this visualization exercise at least once a day for about 10 minutes. Use it when you feel yourself giving in to a craving, or when you're under stress. You'll find that this exercise is a terrific way to rid your body and mind of all kinds of burdens.

Secret #2: Monitor Your Progress

The day before you begin the *6-Day Body Makeover*, weigh yourself on a good scale and take your body circumference measurements with a tape measure. (Refer to the guidelines below.) This is important! Only by weighing and measuring yourself will you be able to compare the exciting changes—in lost pounds and inches—that will take place in your body from Day 1 to Day 6. You may be pleasantly surprised by what you find out. Encouraged by her first experience on the *6-Day Body Makeover*, Cyndie wrote to me: "I followed the [program] to the letter and lost 10 pounds in five days. I've never lost this much this fast before!" Cyndie is now well on her way to her goal weight of 130 pounds, from a start weight of 170 pounds, using my makeover techniques. The only way you're going to be able to track your remarkable progress, as Cyndie did, is to know what your starting weight, your measurements, and your size are before you begin your makeover.

For an accurate before-and-after comparison, always weigh yourself at the same time of day. You can lose a few pounds of water weight overnight and then gain it back during the day. Thus, weighing at the same time every day ensures accuracy. Also, always measure yourself in the same spots and at the same time of the day, making sure the tape measure fits snugly around the body but does not indent the skin areas being measured. As you measure, align the tape measure in a horizontal plane so that it is parallel to the floor. It is best to use a nonelastic tape measure, such as one that is made out of plastic.

Good areas to measure are:

- **Chest:** Directly under your armpits or across the middle of your breasts. Keep the tape measure level around your body.

- **Waist:** Around the smallest part of your waist area.

- **Hips:** Around the widest part of your hip area.

- **Thighs:** Around the largest part of both thighs.

- **Arms:** Extend your upper arm, and wrap the tape measure across the broadest part of your upper arms.

- **Calves:** Around the thickest part of your calves.

In the chart below, record your weight and measurements.

My Progress

Before	Date	After	Date
Weight:		Weight:	
Chest:		Chest:	
Waist:		Waist:	
Hips:		Hips:	
Right thigh:		Right thigh:	
Right arm:		Right arm:	
Right calf:		Right calf:	
Left thigh:		Left thigh:	
Left arm:		Left arm:	
Left calf:		Left calf:	
Size (clothing):		Size (clothing):	

My last word on measuring your progress is a cautionary note on not becoming obsessed with numbers on a scale or inches on a tape measure. There are less tangible but no less significant ways to track your progress: how much better you feel physically, how much more attractive you look, and your increased levels of energy.

Also, consider the value of getting in touch with your body and its needs. For instance, to get rid of body fat, you know you must eat five or six times a day. You know you must cut out processed foods. You know you must eat for your body type and customize around individual medical issues. With the accumulated knowledge you will gain about your body over the next six days, you will see what works for you, and because knowledge is power, you will then have the power to make choices that will keep you healthy and fit for a lifetime. No matter how much you lose, you emerge a winner.

Secret #3: Your Plan for Success

Maybe you've heard it before: If you fail to plan, you plan to fail. It's an old saying, for sure, but the reason these old sayings stick around, quoted over and over again, is because they're true. Planning in advance what you're going to eat over the next six days eliminates any wondering you might do about what to eat when you're hungry—which is often when we make our poorest food choices. In the previous chapter, I mapped out an eating plan for you, telling you exactly what to eat for your body type, and when to eat it. If you're the kind of person who likes to figure out your own custom eating plan, use the tools in this chapter to help you do so.

When you start the *6-Day Body Makeover*, you'll probably find that the foods on your meal plan are tastier than any foods you've had on "diets" in the past. That's because you're eating only the freshest, healthiest foods available. Try not to eat the same vegetables every day, and experiment with the many different ways to prepare your food by taking advantage of the recipes in appendix A. Mapping out a variety of foods and new ways to fix them will prevent boredom from setting in.

On page 117 is a Daily Food Diary to help you plan out your six-day customized eating plan. Simply write in the foods that are appropriate for your body type, along with the amounts. Fill in every slot, including the midmorning and midafternoon snacks. Remember: If you go for long stretches during the day without eating, your body gets the miscue of famine and slows its metabolism, burning calories more slowly.

Once you've mapped out your six-day custom eating plan, you can use it (or the customized eating plan from the previous chapter) to generate a shopping list. A shopping list has many advantages: It helps you decide what to buy before you are tempted by foods in the supermarket, it prevents impulse buying, and it helps you better stick to your custom eating plan. Prior to shopping for the food you need, rid your refrigerator and pantry of what you don't need! Eliminating these foods from your kitchen helps kill cravings and urges to splurge. Stick to healthy foods that are good for you; they can be habit forming!

Keep in mind that while following this program, you'll be eating real food—no processed foods, no packaged foods, no sugar- or salt-laced foods, only clean-burning food that your body can use to take off pounds and inches. Your body was designed to consume and process whole, natural, real foods, and it functions optimally when you provide it with these foods.

DAY 1					
Breakfast	Midmorning	Lunch	Midafternoon	Dinner	PM Snack

DAY 2					
Breakfast	Midmorning	Lunch	Midafternoon	Dinner	PM Snack

DAY 3					
Breakfast	Midmorning	Lunch	Midafternoon	Dinner	PM Snack

DAY 4					
Breakfast	Midmorning	Lunch	Midafternoon	Dinner	PM Snack

DAY 5					
Breakfast	Midmorning	Lunch	Midafternoon	Dinner	PM Snack

DAY 6					
Breakfast	Midmorning	Lunch	Midafternoon	Dinner	PM Snack

That means no diet foods! What people generally don't realize is that diet foods can actually sabotage a weight-reducing diet. This sounds like a contradiction in terms, but it really is true. Instead of saving you a lot of calories, fat, and sugar, many diet foods do just the opposite. Let me give you a few examples to prove my point. Sugar-free cookies, candies, and ice creams often contain just as many calories as their made-with-sugar counterparts. The sugar-free versions many not be made with table sugar, but they are concocted with carbohydrate calories from flour, which can still promote weight gain and high blood sugar, and from sugar alcohols, which can trigger digestive complaints.

Diet shakes and diet bars are just as bad. Many of these products contain as much sugar and fat as a regular candy bar, and you can't lose weight eating candy bars. Further, the protein in these products is not of the best quality and therefore is not utilized by the body as well as egg white, fish, or lean poultry.

Before starting my makeover program, many of my clients had gained anywhere from 10 to 20 pounds drinking just one of these shakes a day as a snack! The reason is that these products are loaded with milk and sugar—both of which will promote weight gain, not weight loss. Using these products to replace even one meal a day forces you to dramatically cut calories. This approach slows your metabolism, and you will regain your weight and usually more. Remember: You have to eat to lose weight—and eat wholesome, natural, clean-burning food.

Low-carb foods are equally problematic. Many of these foods have nearly as many or more fattening calories than their regular-carb versions. Just because a food is designated "low-carb" doesn't mean it's healthy, particularly if it is processed like many of these foods are. Processed foods shut down your metabolism. It's always healthier—and preferable for weight loss—to stick to natural, unprocessed whole foods.

I've generated the following sample customized shopping lists for you. There are five shopping lists, one for each body type. You can make copies of your list, and simply place checkmarks next to the items you need to purchase.

These lists include the approximate amount of the protein you'll need to buy. Meat shrinks when cooked. For each serving of cooked fish, poultry, or meat, buy an extra 2 ounces to allow for shrinkage. Also, you may need more or less of a certain protein, depending on the type you choose for breakfast and other meals. Let your customized eating plan be your guide as to how much protein you need to buy for the next six days.

POULTRY

- ❑ Chicken breast (1½ lbs., uncooked)
- ❑ Turkey breast (2 to 2¼ lbs., uncooked)

FISH (3 to 4½ lbs., uncooked)

- ❑ Cod
- ❑ Flounder
- ❑ Haddock
- ❑ Halibut
- ❑ Red snapper
- ❑ Sea bass
- ❑ Shark
- ❑ Tuna, fresh (3¾ to 4½ lbs. fresh or 36 to 48 oz. canned, no-sodium-added)
- ❑ Other

VEGETABLES & GREENS

- ❑ Asparagus
- ❑ Broccoli
- ❑ Brussels sprouts
- ❑ Cauliflower
- ❑ Celery
- ❑ Cucumber
- ❑ Eggplant
- ❑ Garlic cloves
- ❑ Green and red cabbage
- ❑ Green beans
- ❑ Green onions
- ❑ Greens
- ❑ Jalapeño peppers
- ❑ Leeks
- ❑ Lettuce
- ❑ Mushrooms
- ❑ Okra
- ❑ Onions
- ❑ Parsley
- ❑ Pea pods
- ❑ Pearl onions
- ❑ Peppers
- ❑ Potatoes or sweet potatoes (6 to 12 medium)
- ❑ Radishes
- ❑ Spinach
- ❑ Summer squash
- ❑ Tomatoes
- ❑ Yams
- ❑ Zucchini
- ❑ Other

FRUITS

- ❑ Berries (2 to 3 cups)
- ❑ Grapefruit (2 whole)
- ❑ Lemons
- ❑ Limes
- ❑ Unsweetened applesauce, small jar

BEVERAGES

- ❑ Coffee
- ❑ Distilled water, bottled
- ❑ Sodium-free soda
- ❑ Tea, including herbal tea

HERBS/SPICES/FLAVORINGS

- ❑ Allspice
- ❑ Basil
- ❑ Bay leaves
- ❑ Black pepper
- ❑ Cardamom
- ❑ Cayenne pepper
- ❑ Chili powder
- ❑ Cilantro
- ❑ Cinnamon
- ❑ Coriander
- ❑ Cumin
- ❑ Dill
- ❑ Garlic powder
- ❑ Ginger
- ❑ Marjoram
- ❑ Mrs. Dash or other salt substitute
- ❑ Mustard powder
- ❑ Nutmeg
- ❑ Oregano
- ❑ Paprika
- ❑ Red pepper flakes
- ❑ Rosemary
- ❑ Sesame seeds
- ❑ Tarragon
- ❑ Thyme
- ❑ Turmeric
- ❑ Whole cloves
- ❑ Vanilla extract

STAPLES

- ❑ Apple cider vinegar
- ❑ Balsamic vinegar
- ❑ Chicken broth, sodium- and fat-free
- ❑ Dijon mustard (sodium-free)
- ❑ Herb-flavored vinegar
- ❑ Red cooking wine
- ❑ Rice vinegar
- ❑ Sugar substitute (Splenda, Equal, or stevia)
- ❑ Tomato paste, sodium-free
- ❑ Tomato sauce, sodium-free
- ❑ White cooking wine

EGG WHITES/POULTRY

- ❏ Egg whites (1½ to 2 dozen)
- ❏ Chicken breast (3 to 4½ lbs., uncooked)
- ❏ Turkey breast (2½ to 4½ lbs., uncooked)

FISH

- ❏ Tuna, fresh (2 to 2¼ lbs. fresh or 18 to 24 oz. canned, no-sodium-added)

BEVERAGES

- ❏ Coffee
- ❏ Distilled water, bottled
- ❏ Sodium-free soda
- ❏ Tea, including herbal tea

FRUITS

- ❏ Berries (3 cups)
- ❏ Grapefruit (3 whole)
- ❏ Lemons
- ❏ Limes
- ❏ Unsweetened applesauce, small jar

DRY GOODS

- ❏ Brown rice
- ❏ Long-grain rice
- ❏ Wild rice

VEGETABLES & GREENS

- ❏ Asparagus
- ❏ Broccoli
- ❏ Brussels sprouts
- ❏ Cauliflower
- ❏ Celery
- ❏ Cucumber
- ❏ Eggplant
- ❏ Garlic cloves
- ❏ Green and red cabbage
- ❏ Green beans
- ❏ Green onions
- ❏ Greens
- ❏ Jalapeño peppers
- ❏ Leeks
- ❏ Lettuce
- ❏ Mushrooms
- ❏ Okra
- ❏ Onions
- ❏ Parsley
- ❏ Pea pods
- ❏ Pearl onions
- ❏ Peppers
- ❏ Radishes
- ❏ Spinach
- ❏ Summer squash
- ❏ Tomatoes
- ❏ Zucchini
- ❏ Other

HERBS/SPICES/FLAVORINGS

- ❏ Allspice
- ❏ Basil
- ❏ Bay leaves
- ❏ Black pepper
- ❏ Cardamom
- ❏ Cayenne pepper
- ❏ Chili powder
- ❏ Cilantro
- ❏ Cinnamon
- ❏ Coriander
- ❏ Cumin
- ❏ Dill
- ❏ Garlic powder
- ❏ Ginger
- ❏ Marjoram
- ❏ Mrs. Dash or other salt substitute
- ❏ Mustard powder
- ❏ Nutmeg
- ❏ Oregano
- ❏ Paprika
- ❏ Red pepper flakes
- ❏ Rosemary
- ❏ Sesame seeds
- ❏ Tarragon
- ❏ Thyme
- ❏ Turmeric
- ❏ Whole cloves
- ❏ Vanilla extract

STAPLES

- ❏ Apple cider vinegar
- ❏ Balsamic vinegar
- ❏ Chicken broth, sodium- and fat-free
- ❏ Dijon mustard (sodium-free)
- ❏ Herb-flavored vinegar
- ❏ Red cooking wine
- ❏ Rice vinegar
- ❏ Sugar substitute (Splenda, Equal, or stevia)
- ❏ Tomato paste, sodium-free
- ❏ Tomato sauce, sodium-free
- ❏ White cooking wine

EGG WHITES/POULTRY

- ❑ Egg whites (1½ to 2 dozen)
- ❑ Chicken breast (3 to 4½ lbs., uncooked)
- ❑ Turkey breast (2½ to 4½ lbs., uncooked)

FISH

- ❑ Tuna, fresh (2 to 2¼ lbs. fresh or 18 to 24 oz. canned, no-sodium-added)

VEGETABLES & GREENS

- ❑ Asparagus
- ❑ Broccoli
- ❑ Brussels sprouts
- ❑ Cauliflower
- ❑ Celery
- ❑ Cucumber
- ❑ Eggplant
- ❑ Garlic cloves
- ❑ Green and red cabbage
- ❑ Green beans
- ❑ Green onions
- ❑ Greens
- ❑ Jalapeño peppers
- ❑ Leeks
- ❑ Lettuce
- ❑ Mushrooms
- ❑ Okra
- ❑ Onions
- ❑ Parsley
- ❑ Pea pods
- ❑ Pearl onions
- ❑ Peppers
- ❑ Radishes
- ❑ Spinach
- ❑ Summer squash
- ❑ Tomatoes
- ❑ Zucchini
- ❑ Other

STAPLES

- ❑ Apple cider vinegar
- ❑ Balsamic vinegar
- ❑ Chicken broth, sodium- and fat-free
- ❑ Dijon mustard (sodium-free)
- ❑ Herb-flavored vinegar
- ❑ Red cooking wine
- ❑ Rice vinegar
- ❑ Sugar substitute (Splenda, Equal, or stevia)
- ❑ Tomato paste, sodium-free

BEVERAGES

- ❑ Coffee
- ❑ Distilled water, bottled
- ❑ Sodium-free soda
- ❑ Tea, including herbal tea

DRY GOODS

- ❑ Brown rice
- ❑ Long-grain rice
- ❑ Wild rice

HERBS/SPICES/FLAVORINGS

- ❑ Allspice
- ❑ Basil
- ❑ Bay leaves
- ❑ Black pepper
- ❑ Cardamom
- ❑ Cayenne pepper
- ❑ Chili powder
- ❑ Cilantro
- ❑ Cinnamon
- ❑ Coriander
- ❑ Cumin
- ❑ Dill
- ❑ Garlic powder
- ❑ Ginger
- ❑ Marjoram
- ❑ Mrs. Dash or other salt substitute
- ❑ Mustard powder
- ❑ Nutmeg
- ❑ Oregano
- ❑ Paprika
- ❑ Red pepper flakes
- ❑ Rosemary
- ❑ Sesame seeds
- ❑ Tarragon
- ❑ Thyme
- ❑ Turmeric
- ❑ Whole cloves
- ❑ Vanilla extract

- ❑ Tomato sauce, sodium-free
- ❑ White cooking wine

FRUITS

- ❑ Berries (3 to 7 cups)
- ❑ Grapefruit (3 to 7 whole)

BODY TYPE C CUSTOMIZED SHOPPING LIST

EGG WHITES/POULTRY

- ❏ Egg whites (1 to 2 dozen)
- ❏ Chicken breast (5 to 7½ lbs., uncooked)
- ❏ Turkey breast (1½ to 2¼ lbs., uncooked)

LEAN BEEF (4 to 4½ lbs., uncooked)

- ❏ Arm chuck pot roast
- ❏ Bottom round
- ❏ Eye of round
- ❏ Ground beef, extra lean
- ❏ Round tip (sirloin tip)
- ❏ Tenderloin
- ❏ Top loin (strip loin)
- ❏ Top round
- ❏ Top sirloin

FRUITS

- ❏ Lemons
- ❏ Limes
- ❏ Unsweetened applesauce, small jar

FISH

- ❏ Tuna, fresh (2 to 2¼ lbs. fresh or 18 to 24 oz. canned, no-sodium-added)

BEVERAGES

- ❏ Coffee
- ❏ Distilled water, bottled
- ❏ Sodium-free soda
- ❏ Tea, including herbal tea

DRY GOODS

- ❏ Brown rice
- ❏ Long-grain rice
- ❏ Wild rice

VEGETABLES & GREENS

- ❏ Asparagus
- ❏ Broccoli
- ❏ Brussels sprouts
- ❏ Cauliflower
- ❏ Celery
- ❏ Cucumber
- ❏ Eggplant
- ❏ Garlic cloves
- ❏ Green and red cabbage
- ❏ Green beans
- ❏ Green onions
- ❏ Greens
- ❏ Jalapeño peppers
- ❏ Leeks
- ❏ Lettuce
- ❏ Mushrooms
- ❏ Okra
- ❏ Onions
- ❏ Parsley
- ❏ Pea pods
- ❏ Pearl onions
- ❏ Peppers
- ❏ Radishes
- ❏ Spinach
- ❏ Summer squash
- ❏ Tomatoes
- ❏ Zucchini
- ❏ Other

HERBS/SPICES/FLAVORINGS

- ❏ Allspice
- ❏ Basil
- ❏ Bay leaves
- ❏ Black pepper
- ❏ Cardamom
- ❏ Cayenne pepper
- ❏ Chili powder
- ❏ Cilantro
- ❏ Cinnamon
- ❏ Coriander
- ❏ Cumin
- ❏ Dill
- ❏ Garlic powder
- ❏ Ginger
- ❏ Marjoram
- ❏ Mrs. Dash or other salt substitute
- ❏ Mustard powder
- ❏ Nutmeg
- ❏ Oregano
- ❏ Paprika
- ❏ Red pepper flakes
- ❏ Rosemary
- ❏ Sesame seeds
- ❏ Tarragon
- ❏ Thyme
- ❏ Turmeric
- ❏ Whole cloves
- ❏ Vanilla extract

STAPLES

- ❏ Apple cider vinegar
- ❏ Balsamic vinegar
- ❏ Chicken broth, sodium- and fat-free
- ❏ Dijon mustard (sodium-free)
- ❏ Herb-flavored vinegar
- ❏ Red cooking wine
- ❏ Rice vinegar
- ❏ Sugar substitute (Splenda, Equal, or stevia)
- ❏ Tomato paste, sodium-free
- ❏ Tomato sauce, sodium-free
- ❏ White cooking wine

EGG WHITES/POULTRY

- ❑ Egg whites (1 to 2½ dozen)
- ❑ Chicken breast (3 to 7 lbs., uncooked)
- ❑ Turkey breast (1½ to 2½ lbs., uncooked— can be used in place of egg whites)

LEAN BEEF (5¼ to 7 lbs., uncooked)

- ❑ Arm chuck pot roast
- ❑ Bottom round
- ❑ Eye of round
- ❑ Ground beef, extra lean
- ❑ Round tip (sirloin tip)
- ❑ Tenderloin
- ❑ Top loin (strip loin)
- ❑ Top round
- ❑ Top sirloin

FRUITS

- ❑ Berries (up to 9 cups)
- ❑ Grapefruit (up to 9 whole)
- ❑ Lemons ❑ Limes
- ❑ Unsweetened applesauce, small jar

BEANS

- ❑ Dried beans, any variety
- ❑ Canned beans, low or no sodium, any variety

BEVERAGES

- ❑ Coffee
- ❑ Distilled water, bottled
- ❑ Sodium-free soda
- ❑ Tea, including herbal tea

DRY GOODS

- ❑ Brown rice
- ❑ Long-grain rice
- ❑ Wild rice

VEGETABLES & GREENS

- ❑ Asparagus
- ❑ Broccoli
- ❑ Brussels sprouts
- ❑ Cauliflower
- ❑ Celery
- ❑ Cucumber
- ❑ Eggplant
- ❑ Garlic cloves
- ❑ Green and red cabbage
- ❑ Green beans
- ❑ Green onions
- ❑ Greens
- ❑ Jalapeño peppers
- ❑ Leeks
- ❑ Lettuce
- ❑ Mushrooms
- ❑ Okra
- ❑ Onions
- ❑ Parsley
- ❑ Pea pods
- ❑ Pearl onions
- ❑ Peppers
- ❑ Radishes
- ❑ Spinach
- ❑ Summer squash
- ❑ Tomatoes
- ❑ Zucchini
- ❑ Other

HERBS/SPICES/FLAVORINGS

- ❑ Allspice
- ❑ Basil
- ❑ Bay leaves
- ❑ Black pepper
- ❑ Cardamom
- ❑ Cayenne pepper
- ❑ Chili powder
- ❑ Cilantro
- ❑ Cinnamon
- ❑ Coriander
- ❑ Cumin
- ❑ Dill
- ❑ Garlic powder
- ❑ Ginger
- ❑ Marjoram
- ❑ Mrs. Dash or other salt substitute
- ❑ Mustard powder
- ❑ Nutmeg
- ❑ Oregano
- ❑ Paprika
- ❑ Red pepper flakes
- ❑ Rosemary
- ❑ Sesame seeds
- ❑ Tarragon
- ❑ Thyme
- ❑ Turmeric
- ❑ Whole cloves
- ❑ Vanilla extract

STAPLES

- ❑ Apple cider vinegar
- ❑ Balsamic vinegar
- ❑ Chicken broth, sodium- and fat-free
- ❑ Dijon mustard (sodium-free)
- ❑ Herb-flavored vinegar
- ❑ Red cooking wine
- ❑ Rice vinegar
- ❑ Sugar substitute (Splenda, Equal, or stevia)
- ❑ Tomato paste, sodium-free
- ❑ Tomato sauce, sodium-free
- ❑ White cooking wine

Secret #4: Pre-Prepare Meals for Ease and Convenience

You eat a lot of food on this six-day plan, and if you're as busy as most people are, it is not always easy to get motivated to make meals. You're probably wondering: *How do I find time to cook and fix all of this food?* The answer is amazingly simple: Shop once a week from your shopping list and cook your meals ahead of time, in bulk, once or twice during the six-day period. Think of it this way: It doesn't take any longer to cook four chicken breasts than it does to cook one.

Here are some suggestions for pre-preparing your food that will make meal planning a cinch over the next six days:

- Hard-boil your eggs, store them in the refrigerator, and you'll have egg whites ready to go. Or break fresh eggs, eliminate the yolk, place the whites in a plastic container with a small amount of water, microwave, add pepper, and your breakfast is ready.

- Preslice your fruit and store it in a plastic container in the refrigerator until you're ready to eat it.

- Buy "salad in a bag"—lettuce and greens that are precut for convenience.

- Steam and store your vegetables in the refrigerator; they'll keep for two to three days without losing their freshness. To reheat steamed vegetables, add a bit of water and microwave in a bowl for a few seconds. They'll taste like they've been freshly steamed.

- Bake, microwave, or boil potatoes or sweet potatoes by the dozen. They will keep for a week in your refrigerator as long as they are sealed in a container. To reheat them, simply pop them in the microwave for a minute or less.

- Boil rice ahead of time and store in the refrigerator. It will keep for two to three days before spoiling. Or try the Japanese sticky style of rice; it stays moist and usable longer than other varieties.

- Bake a turkey breast, cover it with a wet paper towel to preserve moisture, and store it in the refrigerator. Reheat your portion in the microwave when you need it for a meal.

- Marinate and grill a dozen chicken breasts on the barbecue, then store them in a plastic container in the refrigerator. When you're ready to eat, pop them in the microwave with a little marinade sauce, and you've got protein anytime. Do the same for lean beef if it's on your custom eating plan.

- Store fish frozen. Season and cook the amount of fish you need for the next six days. Then cut it into right-sized portions and wrap the pieces in individual plastic packets. Put all the packets in a freezer bag to ensure freshness and reheat one in the microwave when you need it. Also, buy plenty of small cans of no-sodium-added tuna to have on hand in a pinch.

Plateau Busters

If you feel like you're not losing weight fast enough, don't get discouraged. Keep following your program. Try any or all of the following plateau busters:

- Increase your exercise, either in duration or in frequency. (Refer to chapter 6 for guidelines.)

- Increase your water intake for a few days. Adequate water intake improves metabolism and may help bring your body back into balance.

- If you've been eating the same thing day after day, including variety in your meals can help. Sometimes the body gets overly accustomed to the same food all the time.

- Review what you've been doing: Have you eaten out? (Food in restaurants is hidden with dietary saboteurs that may disrupt the chemical process involved in burning fat.) Did you eat anything prepared with sugar or salt? Are you eating five to six times a day? Have you skipped meals? Breaking past a plateau actually means eating more food.

The good news: Once you break your plateau, weight loss resumes very quickly!

If you fall off the *6-Day Body Makeover* after a couple of days, don't punish yourself and don't obsess over it. It is not a failure. Think of it as a slip, not a fall. Above all, don't talk yourself into a binge by saying, "I've blown it, so I might as well eat anything I want." That kind of thinking can lead to an all-out eating binge and sabotage your efforts. As the old saying goes, get back on your horse and ride! Start the makeover where you left off.

If you're tempted to slip, do something that doesn't involve food in order to take your mind off your diet. Go for a walk, jog, or run. Read a book. Go to the movies. Do whatever it takes to put yourself in a healthy, motivated frame of mind. The urge to splurge will pass before you know it.

Remember, you are in control. You have the power to make healthful choices and start losing weight again.

To sum up, dropping a dress or pant size in six days is achieved by reprogramming your mind and planning a win–win strategy. The secrets in this chapter are really the tools that make success happen, and you can use them well beyond the six days of this program. They will open up new paths to lifestyle change that can help you reach a lower weight and stay there for life.

CHAPTER 6

Your Fat-Burning Weapon: Long Slow Distance Exercise

Let me tell you about a different but highly effective way to burn fat that breaks all the rules—no sweaty exercise, no endless jumping up and down in a fast-paced aerobics class, no pedal pumping in a grueling Spinning class. In fact, what would you say if I told you that *the harder you work out, the less fat you burn*?

You probably think that sounds crazy—and runs completely counter to everything you've heard or have been taught. But this crazy-sounding statement is actually true. Strenuous exercises such as stair climbing, elliptical machines, aerobic dancing and step classes, rowing machines, kickboxing, and power cycling (Spinning) classes involve the use of certain muscle fibers that expend mostly glycogen (a form of sugar stored in your muscles and bloodstream) for their fuel. In other words, these exercises burn sugar. When your body is burning sugar, it is *not* burning fat.

People once thought that any exercise that didn't have you pounding the pavement or working up a dripping sweat wouldn't help you burn fat. If you weren't running or aerobic dancing your buns off, you weren't going anywhere, and neither was your body fat. No more. Now we know that less-intense exercise is really the secret for shifting your body into a fat-burning mode.

So if you cringe at the thought of intensity-filled workouts, there is a better way to exercise—a method that melts the stored fat on your body without working out so strenuously or becoming a fitness fanatic. It is called *long slow distance exercise*—a form of exercise that includes purposely paced (not intense or strenuous) walking, slow jogging, treadmill exercise, or stationary bicycling, performed 45 to 60 minutes at a stretch. The beauty of long slow distance exercise is that it activates fat burning by creating a demand in your body for more fuel. This way of exercising is actually the most successful way to coerce your body into burning fat and is one of the workout methods I use with all my clients, as well as with the people who appear on *Extreme Makeovers*. Used during the *6-Day Body Makeover*, long slow distance exercise cranks up fat burning and helps you walk or jog off pounds and inches so that you will see a dramatic transformation by the end of this six-day period.

Countless clients have been surprised at how they don't have to kill themselves in the gym or anywhere else with long slow distance exercise. Cary, who used the *6-Day Body Makeover* to get in shape for her 30th high school reunion, told me: "At first I shuddered at the thought of having to exercise. I always hated to sweat! Exercise was always too hard, too demanding, so I never moved a muscle. But I was willing to try long slow distance, and it was tolerable. Then, much to my amazement, I lost 9 pounds on the *6-Day Body Makeover*. I'm sure that long slow distance exercise made all the difference. Now that I realize that I don't have to sweat to lose weight, I enjoy this form of exercise so much more than anything else I've done."

While following the *6-Day Body Makeover*, simply focus on long slow distance exercise because it is one of the most efficient ways to activate rapid fat loss to help you lose one dress or pant size in the allotted six days. But beyond the six days, you'll want to add weight training to your overall exercise routine, particularly to keep losing weight and ultimately to keep that weight off. Although not a component of the *6-Day Body Makeover*, weight training is important to long-term weight control because *over time* it builds metabolically active muscle tissue. The more muscle you have on your body, the more efficient your metabolism is, since muscle burns calories, even at rest. This helps any surplus of fat melt off your body and is among the best ways to keep flab off. Unless you weight train, you can lose an average of ½ pound of muscle each year after the age of 25. But with weight training, even muscle that is often lost to aging can be regained.

When you do weight training or apply some sort of resistance in the form of weights or exercise bands to challenge your muscles, you actually break down muscle cells. Then with rest and proper nutrition, they heal, but become stronger and more shapely as they regenerate. Incorporating weight training into your routine is a part of the deep-seated lifestyle change you must make to be successful at weight control. In chapter 8, you'll learn how to get on a resistance program so that you can ultimately reshape your body, lose additional weight, and keep it off.

The Muscle Fiber Connection

In the past, you've probably exercised your buns off, but without getting very good results. All that huffing and puffing, and you're still having trouble getting into your clothes. I've heard your frustration before—which is why I designed this cardiovascular fitness program of long slow distance exercise so that you can blast away pounds and inches.

There are specific physiological reasons why this form of exercise works so effectively to target body fat, and they have to do with the composition of your muscle. On average, the human body is one-half muscle—voluntary muscle used for movement, smooth or visceral muscle that lines various organs, and cardiac muscle that helps govern the pump action of your heart. They all operate the same general way—by contracting and relaxing. This occurs because the muscle fibers, which are bundles of contracting units that make up the muscle, can shorten their length by 30 to 40 percent.

When you exercise, you use your voluntary muscles, those that move the skeleton's bones in response to the brain's conscious will. There are three types of fibers present in voluntary muscle tissue: fast-twitch fiber, medium- or middle-twitch fiber, and slow-twitch fiber. Depending on your body type, you may have more of one kind than another. Nonetheless, muscle fibers are highly "plastic"; in other words, they can alter their characteristics according to the type of exercise you perform. This means you can make all of these muscle fibers work for you—and mold your physique to the body of your dreams. Let's take a closer look at what I'm talking about.

Fast-Twitch Fiber — The Strength Muscle

When you swing a golf club, lift a barbell, throw a baseball, or sprint, you recruit fast-twitch muscle fibers. These fibers contract quickly, providing short bursts of energy required for these types of explosive movements. This type of muscle fiber does not burn fat. Instead, the primary energy source for fast-twitch muscle fibers is blood sugar stored in the muscle cells themselves, as well as in the blood and liver. Although fast-twitch muscle fiber is the strength fiber, this energy source is quickly depleted, which is why a sprinter must rest after 50 to 100 yards, and a bodybuilder must rest between each set of exercises. In fact, a fast-twitch muscle fiber will give out after about 30 seconds of continuous contraction.

Fast-twitch muscle fiber is dense and hard, giving the body a muscular look. Weight lifters, football players, sprinters, and bodybuilders tend to develop an abundance of fast-twitch fibers in their musculature. If you lift weights for exercise (which I highly recommend), fast-twitch fiber is one of the fibers you'll use to shape, tone, define, and strengthen your body.

Medium- or Middle-Twitch Fiber — The Everyday Muscle

Medium- or middle-twitch fiber is very similar to fast-twitch fiber, in that it is also involved in explosive types of activity. However, it is capable of longer periods of activity and does not have quite the strength capacity of the fast-twitch fiber. When you use many of the cardio machines in the gym, take aerobics classes, or play basketball, you're using middle-twitch fibers. These are movements requiring explosive high-intensity activity but not of the quick, forceful nature of lifting a heavy weight repeatedly for 30 seconds. Like fast-twitch fiber, middle-twitch fiber burns sugar; it does not burn fat. Medium-twitch muscle fiber can be developed through weight-training and body-sculpting exercises.

Slow-Twitch Fiber — The Fat-Burning Muscle

If you've committed yourself to dropping a size in six days, you want to lose as much fat as possible—and do it in the most efficient way you can. That's where slow-twitch fiber comes in. Slow-twitch fiber is your body's fat-reducing fiber. This type of fiber gets most of its energy from burning fat for fuel, in conjunction with oxygen, contracting very slowly but having the ability to endure over extended periods of activity. Recruited when endurance is needed, slow-twitch fiber is very fatigue-resistant, utilized predominantly during the performance of aerobic exercise. This fiber has only a limited ability to increase in size, and as such, little, if any, muscular growth can take place.

Long-distance runners, long-distance cyclists, marathon runners, or any type of endurance athletes tend to develop a greater percentage of slow-twitch fiber. That's why these athletes are generally very thin. They utilize their body fat as fuel, burning it during a process known as the Krebs cycle. Through the Krebs cycle, your body metabolizes fat into energy. But this cycle doesn't kick in until you've done at least 15 to 20 minutes of long slow distance exercise. This creates a slow but steady demand for more energy. The body then taps into its fat stores and combusts that fat for fuel to satisfy the demand. Basically, the goal in long slow distance exercise is to use as much slow-twitch muscle fiber as possible, for as long as possible, so that you can dramatically accelerate the rate at which your body burns fat.

Making It Work: Your 6-Day Workout Program

Okay, now that we've looked at the science behind why long slow distance exercise works, now it's time to make it work for you. To help you get down to a new size, I've designed this workout program to not only help you burn fat but also help you become more fit. Of course, when you use it in conjunction with your customized six-day diet plan, you can expect to see the pounds and inches melt off. Quick results are certainly the best motivation, and the *6-Day Body Makeover* delivers them. But there are many more benefits in store over the long haul: If you make a 100 percent commitment to long slow distance exercise as a lifestyle, it can help normalize your blood pressure, elevate your mood, reduce tension, offset the declining metabolic rate normally associated with aging, and protect you against heart disease. All of these benefits are what I call a mind–body pattern of fitness. They can keep you on track not just with weight control, but with your entire life. Fortifying your mind and your body is an absolute necessity for fitness success.

Ready to finally do it? Keep reading and let's continue your new-you *6-Day Body Makeover*. Here are the steps to making it happen.

Step 1: Choose Your Activity

One of the positive aspects of long slow distance exercise is that you have plenty of options. For optimum fat burning, the best activities include the following:

PACED WALKING

Walking is a do-anywhere activity that anyone can do, and it just happens to be one of the most effective fat-burning workouts there is—as long as you do it rhythmically. I call this Paced Walking, in which you keep your pulse within a certain range for an extended period of time, without much fluctuation, to burn fat (this is explained below). Walking is the perfect choice if you are out of shape or have done little or no cardiovascular exercise in the past.

Some other important tips:

- Wear comfortable clothes; a good pair of sturdy, well-cushioned walking or running shoes; and a watch with a second hand, a stopwatch, or a heart rate monitor.

- Wear reflective clothing if you exercise outside before sunrise or after dark.

- Warm up prior to exercising and make sure you cool down afterward. This helps prevent injury and maximizes the oxygen uptake by your muscles for accelerated fat burning.

- Do not walk on hilly terrain. Stay on flat ground; this ensures that your heart rate stays consistent and steady.

- To minimize the risk of injury, avoid walking on hard pavement such as concrete; stick to softer terrain like grass, footpaths, dirt, or rubber tracks, and so forth.

- Make sure your walking path is safe and well lit, and let other people know your route. Carry a noisemaker or whistle.

- Let your heel strike the ground first, then roll from your heel to the ball of your foot. Push off with the ball of your foot for greater momentum.

- Stop and check your pulse every five to six minutes to stay in your Fat-Burning Zone (which is explained below). If your heart rate is too fast, slow down your pace. If it's too slow, push yourself a little harder.

WALK/JOG

If you're already a walker, now might be a good time to pick up the steam with a walk/jog. This means alternating between a fast walk and slow jog to keep your heart rate where it needs to be. What I've found to be most effective for people who are ready to push a little harder is to walk rhythmically for five minutes, followed by slow jogging for five minutes. Continue this pattern of exercise for 45 to 60 minutes (preceded by a warm-up and followed by a cool-down). A walk/jog is the perfect bridge to the next level of intensity—jogging. Follow the same pointers I've given for walking and for jogging.

SLOW JOGGING

If you've become good at your walking workouts, but the scale never budges, it may be time to cover some new ground with jogging. When you advance to slow jogging, expect to see results very quickly. I have found slow jogging to be the most effective method for fat burning, particularly if you want to begin trimming your hips, thighs, and buttocks.

Even so, jogging is one of the hardest exercises on the musculoskeletal system and can increase the risk of injuries such as twisted and sprained ankles, low back problems, shin splints, knee injuries, and muscle sprains. To reduce these risks, wear proper shoes, stay on soft terrain such as grass, dirt, or rubber tracks, and make sure to warm up first and cool down afterward. Here are some additional guidelines for slow jogging:

- Maintain good posture, with your head and chin up.

- Keep your elbows bent at a 90-degree angle and close to your sides. Let your arms swing backward and forward as you jog.

- Take fairly short strides, letting your heel strike first.

- Monitor your heart rate to make sure you stay in your Fat-Burning Zone.

- Do not jog if you have back, knee, ankle, or foot problems, or any sort of cardio-vascular disease.

TREADMILL

Treadmills provide an ideal way to do your long slow distance walking or jogging indoors, at home, or in a gym. With treadmill exercise, it is easy to keep your pace constant and maintain your heart rate in your Fat-Burning Zone. Also, most treadmills have some cushioning in the tread, which will reduce the impact on your joints. Motorized treadmills are preferable to manual treadmills because they keep the pace steady. Manual treadmills can force you to work too hard. Follow these guidelines for treadmill exercise:

- *Start slow to warm up.* After five or six minutes, step off the treadmill to check your heart rate. To avoid injury, do not try to check your pulse while on the machine. If your heart rate is too slow, crank up the speed on the treadmill. It it's too fast, turn it down.

- *Do not adjust the grade or slope of the treadmill.* Instead, adjust the incline as flat as it will go. Inclined treadmills can place stress on your lower back and may also cause you to work too hard to burn fat.

STATIONARY BICYCLE

A popular means of long slow distance exercise, the stationary bicycle is a good fat burner and overall fitness enhancer. It increases your lower body tone and enhances your aerobic power, provided you exercise consistently in your Fat-Burning Zone. Here are some tips to help you effectively burn fat:

- Use light tension with very little resistance so that the wheels spin easily and you can keep your pulse in your Fat-Burning Zone.

- Adjust your seat height correctly by placing one of the pedals in the fully lowered position. Sit on the bike and extend your leg to the pedal, making sure there's a light bend in your knee. If not, readjust the seat accordingly. Improper seat height can place undue stress on your joints.

- Avoid programs that have you going up and down hills; stay level so that you don't miss out on the fat-burning benefits of stationary bicycling.

- Don't opt for stationary bicycling if you have very large legs, since this form of long slow distance exercise may build up your legs. Choose walking or jogging instead; these activities are more effective for slimming and toning your legs and hips.

- Stationary bicycling can be tough on the hips, lower back, ankles, and knees if you're not accustomed to this form of exercise. If it hurts, don't do it! If you can't adjust the machine to make it comfortable, go back to walking or jogging.

Step 2: Find Your Fat-Burning Zone—and Stay There!

The next important step in setting up your long slow distance exercise program is to determine your Fat-Burning Zone. This is the heart rate at which your body burns fat. If the rate at which your heart is beating is too slow during exercise, your efforts will have little fat-burning effect. If your heart rate is too fast, you'll end up burning sugar that is present in the bloodstream (glucose) and less fat. With higher-intensity exercise, your body needs to acquire fuel quickly in order to keep up with your activity; thus, it draws from sugar stores, since sugar converts more easily to energy than fat does. Your goal, then, is to get your heart rate in the zone that exists between "too slow" and "too fast" so your body will burn proportionally more fat than sugar. Exercising in this zone—your Fat-Burning Zone—gives your body more time to break down stored fat and use it as fuel.

So what is your personal Fat-Burning Zone? One way to find out is to use a common formula for estimating your maximum heart rate; you then calculate a percentage of your maximum to define your Fat-Burning Zone. This zone is commonly defined as 55 to 65 percent of your maximum heart rate. To calculate your Fat-Burning Zone, use the following formula:

- Subtract your age from 220 to find your maximum heart rate. Let's say you're 35 years old. Your maximum heart rate would be 185 beats per minute.

- Multiply your maximum heart rate by 55, 60, or 65 percent to find your Fat-Burning Zone. Using the same example, your Fat-Burning Zone would be 102 (185 x .55), 111 (185 x .60), or 120 (185 x .65).

Ideally, the closer you are to 65 percent, the better. However, if you are very heavy, out of shape, or otherwise deconditioned, you should start at 50 percent of your maximum heart rate. (As you continue exercising aerobically beyond the six-day period, you'll want to gradually work your way up to 65 percent of your maximum.)

If you're "math challenged" and hate arithmetic, use the heart rate chart below. Just find your age, and move across to the column to locate the range you're after.

Heart Rate Chart for Men and Women

Age	55%	60%	65%
18–19	111	121	131
20–21	110	120	130
22–23	109	119	129
24–25	108	118	127
26–27	107	116	126
28–29	106	115	125
30–31	105	114	124
32–33	103	113	122
34–35	102	112	121
36–37	101	110	120
38–39	100	109	118
40–41	99	108	117
42–43	98	107	116
44–45	97	106	115
46–47	96	104	114
48–49	95	103	113
50–51	94	102	112
52–53	92	101	111

Age	55%	60%	65%
54–55	91	100	109
56–57	90	98	108
58–59	89	97	107
60–61	88	96	105
62–63	87	95	104
64–65	86	94	103
66–67	85	92	101
68–69	84	91	100
70–71	83	90	99
72–73	81	89	98
74–75	80	88	96
76–77	79	86	95

Important note: *If you are already in very good cardiovascular condition, you are capable of working at 70 percent of your maximum target heart rate.*

To make sure you're in your ideal fat-burning range while exercising, take your pulse by placing your middle and index fingers on the inside of your wrist. Hold them there until you feel the beating of your heart—that is, your pulse. Once you have it, simply count the beats for 10 seconds (use a watch with a second hand or a stopwatch), then multiply that number by 6 to get your heart rate for a minute. Another option for keeping tabs on your heart rate is to invest in a heart rate monitor, a handy piece of technology that costs between $100 and $300.

If your heart rate is slower than where you should be, speed up. If it's faster, slow down to get back in your Fat-Burning Zone. When in your Fat-Burning Zone, you should be breathing a little harder than usual, but still be able to comfortably carry on a conversation without gasping for air. If you continue to use long slow distance exercise after the *6-Day Body Makeover*, you'll develop a sense of the proper pace for your body and you won't have to check your heart rate so often. Even so, you should continue to check periodically so you can make sure you're burning the maximum amount of fat possible.

When it comes to incinerating fat, the longer you work out, the better! Realistically, you don't start burning much fat until you keep your heart rate in your Fat-Burning Zone for at least 5 to 10 minutes, and you don't start burning fat *rapidly* until you've been in that zone for 30 minutes.

So the central idea of long slow distance exercise is to work out aerobically for a longer duration than normal—45 to 60 minutes—at a lower intensity, maintaining your heart rate in the prescribed zone, in order to activate your slow-twitch muscle fibers and utilize more fat for fuel. During the *6-Day Body Makeover*, you should exercise five times. That should be your goal for maximum results. Here is a suggested workout schedule:

Suggested Long Slow Distance Exercise Schedule

Day	Exercise	Warm-Up + Exercise + Cool-Down
1	Paced Walking, walk/jog, slow jogging, treadmill, or stationary bicycle	45 to 60 minutes
2	Paced Walking, walk/jog, slow jogging, treadmill, or stationary bicycle	45 to 60 minutes
3	*Rest*	
4	Paced Walking, walk/jog, slow jogging, treadmill, or stationary bicycle	45 to 60 minutes
5	Paced Walking, walk/jog, slow jogging, treadmill, or stationary bicycle	45 to 60 minutes
6	Paced Walking, walk/jog, slow jogging, treadmill, or stationary bicycle	45 to 60 minutes

Step 3: Breathe Yourself Thin

Here's something else that may surprise you: You can breathe yourself thin! That's right. A special emphasis on breathing while you exercise can make those pounds come off much faster. Why is this activity so important? Fat is a slow-burning fuel that requires oxygen. If oxygen is delivered to your muscle cells in sufficient quantities, your body can more easily burn fat for most of its fuel requirement. Think of it like this: Just as the fire in your fireplace needs oxygen to burn wood, your body needs oxygen to burn fat. The better oxygenated your body is, the more efficiently fat will burn off your body. When you work your slow-twitch muscle fibers aerobically, which means "in the presence of oxygen," it's like fanning that fire—blowing oxygen into it so that the fire turns hotter and hotter.

With my special Abdominal Breathing technique, you further fan the fat-burning fire in your body as you exercise aerobically in order to speed up your rate of weight loss. Here's how it works:

- As you exercise, inhale deeply through your nose for four steps. Fill your abdomen with air first (your abdomen should rise as it is filled with air); then fill your lungs with air. *Note:* If your belly doesn't rise, you're breathing from your upper chest and getting less oxygen as a result.

- Next, exhale through your mouth for two steps, pushing the air out by contracting your stomach muscles.

- Continue to follow this breathing pattern as you perform your long slow distance exercise. It helps ensure that you get as much oxygen as possible to your muscles, which in turn helps you burn as much fat as possible.

- Do Abdominal Breathing several times before you go to sleep at night, as a stomach-tightening and -toning exercise. This pattern of breathing produces a feeling of calm in your body and helps strengthen what I call the mind–body complex. You'll feel invigorated and energized, plus experience greater stress relief and feelings of inner peace.

As you introduce Abdominal Breathing into your exercise program, you'll be delighted to see your body shed pounds and inches steadily. At first, you'll have to concentrate on mastering this technique, but over time and with continued practice it will become a good-for-you, second-nature habit.

Important: Your Warm-Up and Cool-Down

Before beginning your exercise program, prepare your body for the activity with a proper warm-up. Warming up increases the flow of blood to your muscles and connective tissue, causes a gradual elevation in your heart rate, increases the temperature of your active muscles for a better supply of oxygen, and positively affects the speed of muscular contraction. Basically, the warm-up readies your body for action and reduces the possibility of muscle injury and soreness later.

The best way to warm up for long slow distance exercise is simply to begin your routine, but at a slower, easier pace. For example, if you're doing Paced Walking, start by walking at a deliberately slower pace, just to get your blood pumping. Or if you're doing slow jogging, jog in place. Two to three minutes at this slower pace should provide a sufficient warm-up.

Never neglect your warm-up! Sudden exertion without a gradual warm-up can lead to abnormal heart rate and inadequate blood flow to the heart, along with possible changes in blood pressure, all of which can be dangerous, particularly for older exercisers.

After you've finished exercising, be sure to cool down in order to allow your body time to readjust. Slow down gradually by decreasing the intensity of the activity to bring your body back to its resting state. Take an extra lap around the track, pedal the last five minutes slowly, or walk for five minutes after you've jogged.

Never stop suddenly after exercise. This can cause blood to pool in your muscles, reducing blood flow to your heart and brain. You could faint or experience abnormal rhythms in your heart—both of which could be dangerous.

Special Guidelines for Special Situations

If you have already been exercising on a regular basis without any problems, by all means start out by exercising for 45 to 60 minutes. Other people may have to take it a little more slowly and not start the exercise portion of the program at full blast-off speed. Some of you need to take it slow and let your body gradually adapt to the new stress, particularly if you haven't exercised much in the past, if you're very overweight, or if you're of advanced age. There are several special conditions that may warrant tweaking your exercise prescription. If any of the following situations describe you, please do not take them lightly. Following these guidelines is vital to your overall health and well-being.

If you have a cardiovascular problem or any sort of health problem, get your physician's blessing before you begin an exercise program. If you're approved, have your physician determine your Fat-Burning Zone and the level of intensity that is appropriate for you. Only then should you proceed.

If you are 100 pounds or more overweight, consult with your physician before beginning this program. Find out medically what you can do to start. Many people who are overweight get winded just walking to the mailbox. Carrying extra pounds forces your heart and body to work overtime, and consequently you can reach your Fat-Burning Zone very quickly. Shoot for just 50 to 55 percent of your maximum heart rate and walk for at least five minutes. Slowly add a minute or two to that time, or as much as your body will comfortably allow. Keep adding minutes beyond the six days of this program so that you can begin to incorporate fat-burning exercise into your lifestyle.

If you are out of shape, are 50 pounds or more overweight, and/or are advanced in age, start with 5 to 10 minutes of easy walking or stationary bicycling at 55 percent of your maximum heart rate (but get your doctor's okay first!). Slowly add to that time, as your body becomes more accustomed to exercise. Continue to exercise beyond the six days of this program, gradually adding time to your routine, for optimum fat-burning effectiveness.

If you have done little or no cardiovascular exercise in the past, but are otherwise in good health, start with only 10 to 15 minutes at 55 percent of your maximum as your Fat-Burning Zone. Add as many minutes as feels comfortable and doable to you. Beyond the six days of the program, work toward increasing your time to 45 minutes. Then slowly increase your prescribed heart rate in 5 percent increments until you reach 65 percent of your maximum. That way, you'll keep your body in a fat-burning mode each time you exercise.

If you are in reasonably good shape, and 50 pounds or less overweight, start with 20 to 30 minutes at 60 percent of your maximum. Slowly add 5 to 10 minutes to your time as you are able and as you become aerobically more fit. Eventually, work your way up to

45 minutes to an hour per session. At the same time, shoot for increasing your intensity to 65 percent of your maximum in order to reach your Fat-Burning Zone.

Listen to your body! The mantra *no pain, no gain* is a myth. You *will* benefit from a sensible, pain-free, moderate workout program like the long slow distance exercise program I'm recommending for the *6-Day Body Makeover*—and you will blast away body fat. Certainly, exercise should require some effort, but it should not cause pain or discomfort. In fact, if you experience real pain, your body is telling you to stop exercising, so you had better listen to that warning message. If you continue to feel pain during an exercise, stop and do not resume until you can exercise painlessly.

The general muscle soreness that comes after exercising is another matter altogether. It usually indicates that you're not warming up sufficiently or that you are working out too hard or too long. Sore muscles should not discourage you from exercising or make you stop, but they should force you to slow down.

Keep in mind that the possibility of injury is much less with long slow distance exercise than with very intense aerobic exercise that is high impact in nature. High-impact exercise can produce injuries to shins, calves, lower back, ankles, and knees because of the repetitive, jarring movements of the routines. You'll be much more likely to continue to exercise as a lifestyle if you know you won't be sidelined by painful injuries.

Make It Fun

For long slow distance exercise to be maximally effective for fat loss over the next six days, you must do it four to five times during this short makeover period. But if you're like many people, you probably get bored to tears doing a repetitive activity for 45 minutes to an hour. Here are some ways to avoid boredom while performing long slow distance exercise:

- Use a lightweight portable stereo with headphones to listen to your favorite music, books on tape, or *Body Makeover* motivational audiotapes and CDs (see appendix C for information) while you're walking or jogging outdoors. *Caution:* Make sure you can still hear traffic noises. Ignoring what's going on around you can be risky.

AVOID THESE WORKOUTS!

Surprise: Some of the most popular workouts that are effective for cardiovascular fitness are not effective for burning fat. If you really want to burn fat, stick to long, slow, rhythmic workouts such as Paced Walking, slow jogging, a walk/jog, treadmill exercise, or stationary bicycling. Any exercise that has you working too strenuously burns sugar, not fat. A number of these are listed below.

Stair climbing	Circuit training (with weights or machines)
Elliptical machines	Climbing machines (or vertical climbing walls)
Aerobic dancing	Rowing machines
Aerobic step classes	Martial arts
Kickboxing	Boxing
Stair-step machines	Power cycling (Spinning-type classes)

- Watch television while pedaling on a stationary bicycle or walking on a treadmill. Or listen to music, motivational audiotapes, or CDs. If your equipment has a reading rack, read a book or a magazine.

- Change the scenery. If you get bored by your treadmill workout, take a walk outdoors instead.

- Vary your path. If you walk or jog outdoors on the same route every day, consider changing your path to alleviate the sameness.

- Find a "makeover buddy." Recruit a friend or friends to do the *6-Day Body Makeover* with you—including the long slow distance exercise program. You can support one another, help each other when one of you wants to quit, and be inspired by each other's success and progress. Exercising with a buddy is motivating and provides the support you need to see the program through. Plus, it can make the next six days fun!

Food and Fitness

The foods you're eating on the *6-Day Body Makeover* are meant not only to trigger weight loss, but also to energize your body for exercise. On the days that you perform your long slow distance workout, *you must eat one of your allotted carbohydrates prior to exercising.* Remember, carbs are your body's number one food fuel. To push through your workout, your body needs that caliber of fuel. In addition to the protein your meal already contains, add the following carbohydrates *if* your meal does not already contain them:

- If you're a Body Type A, eat a baked potato or yam or 1 cup of oatmeal plus a banana prior to exercising.

- If you're a Body Type B, eat cooked rice (in your serving size), a yam, or large apple prior to exercising.

- If you're a Body Type C, eat cooked rice (in your serving size) or a large apple prior to exercising.

- If you're a Body Type D, eat cooked rice (in your serving size) prior to exercising.

- If you're a Body Type E, eat cooked rice or beans (in your serving size) or 1 cup of oatmeal prior to exercising.

Note: If you find that these additions to your meal make you uncomfortably full, then eat the protein and cut the carbohydrate in half. For example, a female type A would eat *at least* 2 oz. protein, ½ cup oatmeal, and half a banana.

If you tend toward low blood sugar, carry an extra carbohydrate with you, such as a Clif Bar. Eat it if you feel lightheaded or dizzy or you experience other symptoms associated with low blood sugar. Don't eat it if you don't need it.

Also, carry water with you, and drink!

Use long slow distance exercise to become more active and fit. This one small change in your activity level adds up to big results in terms of your fat burn, fitness, and endurance. By the end of the next six days, you'll clearly see why this form of exercise is worth the effort—and you'll be very proud of what you've accomplished and how great you look.

CHAPTER 7

6-Day Body Makeover *Tips from A to Z*

There's no question about it: The *6-Day Body Makeover* is an accelerated, aggressive weight-loss program. So if you want aggressive weight loss—and want to reach your goal of losing a whole dress or pant size in six days—then you've got to be aggressive with your willpower as well, and that means no slipping off the plan. In this chapter, I've included 26 stick-to-it tips and reminders, from A to Z, that make this possible. Many of these suggestions came from people just like you who have used the *6-Day Body Makeover* and my other makeover programs to get the body they wanted.

Aerobic Activity

Never neglect your long slow distance routine! This is one of the best and most efficient forms of cardiovascular exercise to rewire and rev up a slow metabolic rate, plus burn the maximum amount of body fat for fuel during the actual time of exercise. There's more, though: Your metabolism can stay in swing for up to 24 hours after you do your long slow distance routine. Try to do it five times over the next six days, at least

45 minutes each time (unless certain precautions listed in chapter 6 apply to you). If you're not seeing results, adding another 15 minutes to the routine will not only burn more fat but also speed up your metabolism so you burn more fat all day long.

And that's still not all: Aerobic activity stirs up levels of feel-good chemicals in your body called endorphins. They help boost your mood, ease stress, and generally make you feel pumped up mentally. That's a good state of mind to be in while you're doing the *6-Day Body Makeover*.

Beverages

Most people normally don't drink a lot of water, preferring instead soda, sugary coffee drinks, and juices. You definitely want to stay away from fruit juices. A small glass of orange juice is equal to half a dozen or more whole oranges. Six oranges at one sitting aren't on anyone's plan! Also, because the fiber has been removed, fruit juices are almost instantly converted to sugar in your body. While following the *6-Day Body Makeover*, **don't** drink:

- Milk or dairy products (including fat-free dairy products)
- Powdered or dried coffee creamers (even if they're fat-free)
- Fruit and vegetable juices
- Health food shakes or concoctions
- Alcoholic drinks and nonalcoholic wines or beers
- Sports drinks (unless your physician specifies them for low blood pressure, arrhythmias, or other concerns)

All of these beverages are loaded with calories and/or simple sugars and have the ability to slow your metabolism and dramatically reduce weight loss. Water is the best fluid for your body. You wouldn't put soda into your steam iron or car radiator, right? There's no substitute for water, so stick to the basics: water, water, water, and more water.

But if you do require more variety, you may supplement your water intake with other permissible beverages, which are listed below. So during the *6-Day Body Makeover*, in addition to water, **do** drink:

- Iced tea (no sugar added, but a sugar substitute such as Splenda or Equal is fine)
- Lemonade made from fresh lemons and sugar substitute
- Black coffee or tea (including herbal tea)
- Low- or no-sodium sparkling water (beware of club soda, which is usually loaded with sodium)

Creativity

Be adventuresome and try new ways of preparing and cooking your food in order to prevent the dual diet killers—boredom and repetition—from setting in. Both may sabotage your efforts. I've found that people who are the most successful at losing weight introduce a variety of healthy recipes into their meal plans. With a little bit of creativity, you'll find that you can adapt many of your family's favorite foods into fat-burning recipes that fit perfectly into your custom eating plan.

Feel free to incorporate onions, garlic, green or red peppers, fresh jalapeños, chives, tomatoes, and other vegetables into recipes to add rich flavors and make delicious meals your family will love. If you see a recipe for chicken that sounds great or find Grandma's famous meat loaf recipe, try adapting it to fit on your plan. Remember, ground turkey or chicken can replace ground beef in almost every recipe if your body type doesn't respond well to red meat.

Do whatever you need to do, within the guidelines of the *6-Day Body Makeover*, to keep your food enjoyable, including trying the many makeover recipes in appendix A. Being creative with cooking and food preparation plays a key role in your success.

Defeat Cravings

When cravings hit or you're tempted to go off the program, substitute a nonfood activity for eating. Do your exercise routine, take a hot bath, manicure your nails, read a good novel, visit a friend, do some household work—anything that will distract you from eating. Engaging in any activity that competes with eating, or is incompatible with it, will fend off cravings in a hurry. The more you practice this tip, the easier it becomes to ride the wave of a craving.

Energy

If you're afraid that losing weight so quickly will leave you draggy and tired, don't worry another second. True, many quick-weight-loss "diets" do trigger feelings of fatigue because they cut valuable energy-producing foods from the diet, such as carbohydrates and vitamins and minerals (which are catalysts in the body for producing energy). The *6-Day Body Makeover* is an exception, however. You're eating a balanced array of foods, including carbohydrates, and eating a lot of food. What's more, you'll be losing pounds of fat. Weight loss normally helps people become reinvigorated. There is no reason that this program should leave you feeling anything but energized and revitalized.

In the rare event that you do feel fatigued, check your blood pressure. If it's low (90/60 or lower), add some salt to your diet. Or you may need additional carbohydrates if your fatigue is brought on by hypoglycemia. See appendix B for more information on how to tweak your eating plan for special medical conditions.

Family Food Fights

If you're the only family member following the *6-Day Body Makeover,* expect to run into opposition from nondieting folks who may want foods that aren't on your custom eating plan. Here's my solution to this all-too-common conflict: If you must buy other foods for your family, at least buy food products and brands you don't like. Example: If chocolate chip cookies have been your downfall in the past, buy your kids vanilla wafers or some other kind of cookie you don't like. Keep in mind, too, that kids can get all the junk food they want (unfortunately) while they're away from home, so why even have it in your house? You're not depriving your children of anything by not having junk food around; rather, you're helping them become healthier, and that's a wonderful gift.

Give Away Your Large Sizes

Get rid of those larger sizes hanging in your closet, or at least put them in storage. Keeping them around keeps you locked in a fat mind-set and undermines your motivation to reach, and stay at, a smaller, healthier size.

Heroes

One of the most inspirational and motivating moves you can make right now is to listen to success stories of people who have been able to lose weight—the same goal you're trying to achieve. I strongly suggest that you read about or listen to others who have done what you wish to accomplish. There are a number of sources for this information, all readily accessible, including www.provida.com (click on "Success Stories") and www.body makeover.com (click on "Testimonials").

Insulated Cooler

If you're just starting the *6-Day Body Makeover,* you're probably looking for tips to make it easier to eat all your meals and snacks, especially if you work in an office or anyplace where cooking is not an option. Many of my makeover clients report that the simplest answer is the best: an insulated cooler to keep foods hot or cold. For keeping foods cool and fresh, use "blue ice" or other freezable cooling agents. The cooler doesn't have to be big; there are a great variety of sizes and shapes available, so you can easily find one that fits your lifestyle and your budget.

Join Up with Others

If you have a very hard time staying motivated, find a makeover partner to do the program with you—be it a spouse, parent, friend, or sibling. You can support one another, help each other through the next six days, and be inspired by each other's success. Plus, it can make the whole experience much more fun. Scientific research shows that dieting with a partner can be a very powerful part of weight-loss success. Also, consider starting your own *6-Day Body Makeover* Club with other caring people who help one another succeed.

In addition, through www.provida.com, I have established a 24-hour support community where you can link up online with people who have used the *6-Day Body Makeover* to drop a size, plus thousands of other people who have lost hundreds of pounds. This support community has 100,000 members (and growing) and includes everything from general discussion groups to specific forums based on your needs. You can always find someone to be your "online makeover buddy" and make sure you succeed.

Keep Your Daily Food Diary

Keeping your daily food diary makes you conscious of exactly what you're supposed to eat every day on the plan. Most people go about their day totally unaware of how much they're really eating and how many calories they've racked up; then they wonder why they packed on so many pounds! Your daily food diary is an integral part of planning ahead for success. Know what you're going to eat so that you're less tempted to deviate from your custom eating plan.

Lifestyle Change

Even though you're undertaking this program for only six days, think of what you're doing as a catalyst for long-term lifestyle change: an active life that includes regular exercise; a life of healthy eating that includes fruits, vegetables, wholesome carbohydrates, and lean proteins; and a life in which you care about having a healthier, naturally beautiful body that's yours for keeps. Whereas before your lifestyle made you fat, now your lifestyle will keep you lean and fit.

In the next chapter, you'll learn more about how to maintain these lifestyle changes and to keep going if you need to lose more weight. The bottom line, however, is about sticking to the basics: eating five to six times a day, always a protein with a carbohydrate; avoiding processed foods; staying away from sugar, salt, and fats (oil, butter, and so on); and keeping your body trim and fit with regular exercise.

Once you change your body so dramatically in just six days—and you look so fabulous—you're sure to inspire your family members and friends with your new look. They'll want to make the same lifestyle changes you've made. You may end up being a role model to others because of what you've accomplished.

Mini-Goals

An ancient Chinese proverb states: "A journey of a thousand miles starts with one step." Dropping one whole size in six days is a journey, even though it's a short one. Your mini-goals are the steps you take each day to get to the weekend—slimmer, trimmer, and able to fit into a smaller size. This wise proverb is the idea behind setting and keeping *mini-goals*—anything that you think is important to keep you going from day to day. You set them each day. Sticking to anything for a single day is a cinch. You don't have to think about doing the program for six days. Instead you concentrate on *today*. When you take it a day at a time, it becomes incredibly easy. And before you know it, you're one size smaller by Friday.

Seeing yourself achieve your mini-goals will keep you excited and feeling positive about yourself. Your mini-goals will ensure that you experience the progress you're making and prevent you from backsliding. A mini-goal can be anything that helps you stay focused on what you want to achieve in a single day of the program:

- *Today I will stick to my eating plan 100 percent.*
- *Today I will do my long slow distance exercise.*
- *Today I will drink all 12 glasses of water.*
- *Today I will prepare my meals for the next six days.*
- *Today I will plan my meals for the program by filling out my food diary.*

Whatever your mini-goals are, I suggest that you write them down and post them where you can see them. Recording your mini-goals on paper or in your computer drives home the need for doing them.

Never Let Yourself Go Hungry

If you eat the required five to six meals a day on the *6-Day Body Makeover*, you'll never let yourself get hungry—something that's critical to weight loss. Eating those well-spaced-out meals will prevent hunger pangs and the overeating that often accompanies them. It also keeps insulin and blood sugar levels more constant and stable, so your body doesn't go into a fat-storing mode. That's why I must repeat: *Don't skip meals!* Skipping meals will not speed up your weight loss, but will in fact stop the *6-Day Body Makeover* from working. You must eat all the food on your customized eating plan in order for it to work, in order to keep your metabolism burning at a constant, steady pace.

Organize with Technology

Use a calendar, alarm, or organizer program to remind you to drink your water or eat your snacks and meals. Calendar programs such as those available with Microsoft Outlook Express and other e-mail programs can automate this process easily. If you use a handheld computer, use it to keep track of everything you eat, all your water, and your exercise schedule. If you're not at a computer most hours of the day, consider setting an alarm clock or wristwatch with a reminder feature to do the same. Even the alarm feature on your cell phone will do the trick.

Pamper Yourself

Ever since Narcissus in Greek mythology first gazed at his face in a pool of water, humankind has been obsessed with appearance. That's not an altogether negative behavior pattern. Psychological research shows that improved appearance can enhance your self-esteem (how you value and accept yourself for who you are), banish social insecurities, and favorably influence the way others treat you. When you make the right moves to improve your appearance, you bolster your ego and begin to see yourself in a better light.

What's more, pampering treatments—a facial, makeup application, a soothing massage—provide a nurturing touch that is important to your psychological well-being.

There is such a strong appearance/self-esteem connection that I recommend to everyone, men and women, starting the *6-Day Body Makeover* that they pride themselves on how they look. Changes can include having a new hairdo or haircut, getting a sexy new makeup look, or having a facial or a body-sloughing treatment. Even a manicure has an amazing ability to make you feel confident, since hands are such an important means of communication. When your nails are well groomed, you send a message to people that you're competent and have it together.

Transforming the new you definitely goes beyond losing a dress or pant size. There's nothing better than feeling beautiful or handsome to help you shake off sagging motivation to lose weight and to psych you up over the next six days. Promise yourself that while you're working on your diet and exercise program, there will be no more less-than-best moments in your appearance.

Quiet Your Stress

Overeating in response to stress is a huge obstacle to successful weight control. Stress will induce you to eat more than practically anything else will, since eating is often an outlet for relieving pent-up tension or, for many people, a way of avoiding dealing with whatever is stressing them out. In fact, food can be as comforting as a drug, and for many people just as addicting.

When you're under stress, your body churns out two stress hormones, cortisol and adrenaline, which under normal circumstances help you handle stress. If that stress goes unresolved, however, those hormones stay elevated. Cortisol, in particular, isn't metabolized well under these conditions, and when it's in constant circulation it tends to have a fat-accumulating effect, especially in the abdominal region of the body. This type of fat has often been called "stress fat" because it is formed by high levels of stress-induced cortisol in the body. Other damaging effects occur, too, when your body is flooded with stress hormones: a racing heart, increased blood pressure, back pain, headache, or serious illness.

Whether caused by work pressures, financial troubles, relationship difficulties, job loss, or chronic illness, stress is a fact of everyone's life, so don't expect it to miraculously vanish from yours anytime soon. The key to getting it under control so that you don't lose control of your eating is to take anti-stress measures and make them an ongoing part of your lifestyle so that you learn to deal with stress in a healthy manner.

Important caveat: I generally don't recommend that you begin any of my makeover programs during a time of *severe* stress. Rather, I advise people to work on their emotional problems before making wholesale changes to their diets. Even so, there are anti-stress measures already built into the *6-Day Body Makeover,* as well as my other makeover programs. For example:

- *Eating breakfast.* This ignites your metabolism in the morning and fuels your brain to get focused and stay alert. That way, you can better problem-solve your way out of stressful situations and encounters. Having a good breakfast also fights fatigue and counters possible stress eating later in the day.

- *Eating natural foods.* The foods you eat on the *6-Day Body Makeover,* especially fresh fruits and vegetables, are abundant in vitamins, minerals, and antioxidants—all nutrients that naturally combat stress by keeping your immune system strong and resilient.

- *Multiple meals.* Eating frequently every two to three hours provides a constant stream of fuel to your body that keeps stress levels down and energy levels up. More meals doesn't mean fattening snacks, however. Natural, complex carbohydrates (the so-called slow carbs) combined with protein work best to blunt the stress response, boost energy, and prevent brain fatigue.

- *Exercise.* Of all the methods available to relieve stress, exercising may be the most effective and the easiest to do—for three important reasons. First, exercise increases certain brain waves involved in relaxation. Second, it increases the secretion of endorphins in the brain—natural chemicals that give you a feeling of happiness and tranquility. Exercising also boosts confidence and self-esteem, two qualities important to stress control. Third, exercise acts to distract you from the stressors in your life. It's difficult to worry about the problems you face each day when you're working out and concentrating on your exercise routine.

Here are some other anti-stress measures to consider to help you overcome stress eating:

- *Triggers.* Identify stressors that cause you to turn to food. What turns you into an emotional basket case? Your kids? Job tensions? Tight deadlines? The key is to problem-solve in order to control the stressors that cause you to overeat or binge. If your kids keep you stressed out, then you may have to learn better family-management skills, or have grandparents take them off your hands periodically so that you get a break. If you're tense at work, this may require talking to your boss about accommodating whatever is stressful, whether it's long hours, problems with co-workers, or tight schedules or deadlines. You may have to learn to put more balance in your life, so that you can have time for fun, relaxation, and spiritual fulfillment—all life choices that help counteract the effects of stress. The point is: Be active and involved in seeking solutions for stress. This will give you much-needed control over your life—and your eating.

■ *Perception.* Unless you think something is stressful, it will not normally trigger a stress response or the likelihood that you'll run to the refrigerator or pantry for cover. That's why of all mental approaches to life, perception is the most critical. How you size up a situation determines your response to it. Some people become absolutely unglued at life's intrusions, while others use them as an opportunity to shine. Which are you? Think about how your perceptions may heighten your stress response and make stress worse than it really is, then work to modify those perceptions so that you don't turn every incident into a catastrophe.

■ *Healing downtime.* Allow for time to de-stress by practicing relaxation. For some people, this can mean listening to music, reading an enjoyable book, exercising, or practicing meditation. True relaxation induces physical and mental calm, during which the body can eliminate toxins and waste products, replenish fuel stores in muscles and in the bloodstream, and restore energy. Cortisol levels also decline during periods of relaxation. Your mind, body, and spirit all need periodic time-outs to relax and restore. Find time to incorporate relaxation into your daily schedule. Doing so will help you stay more relaxed during the day so that when stress hits, you're less likely to overreact.

Reward Yourself

Doing a good job or achieving a goal customarily deserves a reward. But customarily, the reward amounts to food (you know the drill: "Let's go out to dinner to celebrate"). Rewarding yourself after achieving a perfect six days on the *6-Day Body Makeover* should be a part of your program, but so should rewarding yourself *daily*. This means, for example, that every time you go an entire day and eat every meal on your plan, you've met your goal for that day. So give yourself a reward! This is a supereasy way to give yourself continuous positive feedback for your new dedication to eating right. Of course, your rewards should be of a nonfood nature. For instance, reward yourself with a facial or a massage. Treat yourself to a movie, play, or concert. Buy yourself a new CD or DVD. Schedule a weekend trip. Even some extra sleep or relaxation on the weekend can be a great incentive. Rewards can be simple and inexpensive, too. One of my clients, Anna, puts a gold stick-on star on her wall calendar every day she eats on the plan. The important thing is to give yourself positive feedback every day.

You might want to take an attractive goal-sized outfit and hang it on the wall in your house as an incentive. Then every day you'll be reminded that by making the right choices throughout the day, you can reach that goal. When you lose a clothing size, as you will on the *6-Day Body Makeover*, that outfit will be your reward. Whatever you choose, reward yourself with something that will keep your enthusiasm high.

It's a good idea to write down what your rewards will be, so you have something to look forward to. These rewards—these "carrots on a stick"—will keep you going. So choose those carrots now!

Sidestep Saboteurs

Once you decide to follow the *6-Day Body Makeover*, don't expect everyone in your life to go along with your decision. Your friends and relatives may not understand your determination to drop a size by next weekend. They may feel jealous or threatened by your efforts, and in response they may try to tempt you with goodies, or feel hurt when you reject a piece of homemade pie.

If you're faced with saboteurs, there are ways you can gracefully sidestep their inducements of food. Straightforward honesty, for example, works in most cases: "The dessert is beautiful, and I know you put a lot of time into it. But I'm trying to slim down and eat in a more healthy fashion, and I know you'll want to support me in that."

If your social life typically revolves around food, suggest to your friends that you try something that's not so food-focused the next time you get together, such as going to a concert, attending a play, visiting a museum, or making your own pottery at a ceramics store. Ask your friends to understand if you turn down dinner this week.

Be assertive. If someone continually tries to "force-feed" you with junk, stand up for yourself. Be polite, but firm: "No thank you. I don't need it."

Time Management

The biggest excuse people give for not exercising is "I don't have time." The fact that you're doing the *6-Day Body Makeover* already says that you're committed to dropping a size and losing pounds and inches along with it. Remember that this program is different: You don't have to spend two hours at the gym every day to see results. But you do have to make time for doing your long slow distance routine for 45 to 60 minutes four to five times over the next six days. No matter how busy you are, do anything you can to make time for this routine. Here are some suggestions to help you:

- Get up early to exercise, when your workout time is least likely to be interrupted by other things. Or ask your spouse to watch the kids for 45 minutes every evening so you can walk.

- Walk on a treadmill while watching TV with your family.

- Block out time on your calendar for exercise, just as you would with any scheduled appointment. Guard that time slot; it is your time to take care of yourself.

- Put exercise high on your priority list. If it's number 10 or 16 on your list, you won't do it. Move it up the list!

Keep in mind, too, that every minute you do your long slow distance routine, past the first 30 minutes, you're burning fat off your body at an incredible rate! This is another activity where you won't know if you have time to do it until you start. At first, 45 minutes may seem like a long time, but long slow distance exercise will dramatically increase fat loss and improve nearly every aspect of your life. It is the best and easiest way to increase energy, reduce stress, and just plain make you feel better.

Use Your Mirror

In addition to your scale and a tape measure, your mirror can be an effective tool for evaluating your progress, even over the next six days. The mirror doesn't lie and is often more reliable than the fluctuating number of pounds that register on the scale. If it looks like the program has stalled for a day or two, based on what your scale says, your spirits may sag, and in some people this can lead to bingeing. Women, in particular, occasionally have seesaw hormonal swings that can send the scales soaring one day and dipping down the next. So don't be afraid to look in your mirror to check how you look and see where the fat is burning off. At the same time, you can give yourself loving, positive affirmations about your body, how good you feel, and the progress you're making toward looking your best. And you don't have to look at yourself in the buff, either. Use the mirror to check how well your clothes are fitting and how great you look in them. If improving your appearance is one of your primary motivations for doing the *6-Day Body Makeover,* then the mirror is a great way to notice that improvement.

Variety

We require variety in our diets; in fact, we're all born with a need for it. The latest research says that unless we indulge this innate requirement for variety, our health will be jeopardized. People who eat the least varied diets are most likely to suffer from heart disease and cancer because they do not obtain the full array of vitamins, minerals, and phytochemicals available from a broad range of foods. All of these naturally occurring nutrients play a vital role in our health.

Limiting the number of different foods you eat while trying to lose weight and inches is not only a nutritional disaster, but also sets up a no-win situation—in two major ways, according to other research. First, the more monotonous your diet is, the more likely you are to cave in to food cravings. You know exactly what I'm talking about if you've ever gone on the cabbage soup diet, the grapefruit diet, the rice diet, or some other single-food diet. After a few days, there's only so much cabbage, grapefruit, or rice you can choke down. Pretty soon, you're off that diet and gobbling down any food in sight because you've gotten so bored with a food you've been eating meal after meal, day after day. When this monotony effect kicks in, your weight-loss efforts are doomed.

Second, people who eat a greater variety of plant foods (fruits, vegetables, and whole grains) weigh less than people who limit their food choices. That's because they're eating foods that help them feel full, satisfied, and more energized.

The preparation of delicious, great-tasting food plays a huge role in your success— and helps you stick to the six-day program without getting bored or tired of the foods you'll be eating. The more variety you have, the less likely you are to deviate from your customized eating plan, and that means you will easily reach your goal of a smaller size in just six days. Use as many of the recipes in appendix A as you can to add variety to your eating plan.

Water

Now, don't go skipping off to the next chapter, proclaiming that you're tired of me harping on water! For this program to work, you must drink your twelve 8-ounce glasses, or 100 ounces, of water every day. Water is vital to weight loss: Drinking water and then eliminating it from your system revs up your metabolism and prevents fluid retention. Drinking enough water daily can even blunt your appetite by giving you that "full" feeling, so you're less likely to give in to food temptations. Some people can actually lose weight just by increasing their water intake.

One of my clients, Dottie, sent in this great trick that makes it easy to keep track of your water intake. Take a standard 20-ounce sports bottle and put five rubber bands around it. Every time you drink a bottleful, take off a rubber band. When the last band is gone, you've drunk all your water. Another client, Claire, uses a slight variation on this tactic: She puts on five bracelets at the beginning of the day, and takes one off every time she finishes a 20-ounce bottle of water.

X-Rated Additives

There are additives in foods that will jeopardize your efforts at weight loss and weight control. That's why I advise all my clients to stay away from additive-laced prepackaged foods while following the *6-Day Body Makeover*. Topping the list of food additives that undermine your weight and your diet are sodium, sugars, corn syrup (including high-fructose corn syrup), dextrose, hydrogenated fats, starch and modified starch (used in many foods as thickening agents), and the flavoring agent monosodium glutamate (which has recently been linked scientifically to obesity). These additives and the foods that contain them play havoc with your body chemistry.

You want your body to break down the food you feed it as quickly as possible. When you add preservatives and chemicals, your body chemistry gets sluggish and lethargic, and you stop losing weight. So remember: Buy only the freshest foods you can, and prepare them yourself.

Yo-Yo Dieting Dangers

You'll learn more about maintaining your weight loss and your new clothing size as soon as you turn the pages to the next chapter, but for now, understand that your new way of eating, which you'll want to maintain for a lifetime, is an effective way to prevent yo-yo dieting because it keeps your metabolism constantly charged up. Yo-yo dieting, in which dieters lose and gain weight in cycles, is something you'll want to avoid. One newly discovered reason is that it can make you more susceptible to infections, according to new research that looked into the practice (known as weight cycling in the scientific world). Among women who had lost significant amounts of weight at least five times, their "natural killer cell" function dropped by 30 percent. These cells are a vital part of your body's disease-fighting army against viruses, such as the common cold, viral pneumonia, herpes, and human papillomavirus, which can cause cervical cancer. The message here is that yo-yo dieting is dangerous! What you need is a weight-control program that has a sustainable result, and is not a temporary fix. I'll show you how to make that happen when we get to the next chapter.

Zip Up

Finally, here's more encouragement you've been waiting to hear: I hope that outfit you've had your eye on is hanging in your closet, because before long you'll be wearing that smaller size and be special-occasion trim. If you follow this program to the letter and use the tips here, you'll lose enough weight to zip into clothes that are one whole size smaller than you are wearing at this very instant!

By now, you know that there are plenty of techniques for getting in shape that you never knew of before. So keep aiming high, just as you have been, and I'll show you how to achieve longer-term weight-loss goals so that you'll never look back on the way you used to look!

CHAPTER 8

The Seventh Day and Beyond:
What to Do Next

Your six days are up!

Congratulations: You did it. You completed the *6-Day Body Makeover*.

Right now, look at yourself in the mirror, wearing your new outfit that is one size smaller than you used to wear. If you stuck with the program, you're looking and feeling fabulous in your new smaller-sized dress, pants, or other outfit. You're ready to show the new, smaller you to the world. Count on getting plenty of compliments this weekend on how great you look. Everyone will wonder: How did you do it? They'll want to know your secret.

I realize that you undertook the *6-Day Body Makeover* to drop a clothing size, get in shape for a special occasion, take off pounds and shed inches fast, jump-start your weight loss, or smash past a plateau. But I also know that you also undertook this makeover to stay at your new size, to keep that weight off, or to start losing even more weight. Now it's the seventh day, and you'd like to know what to do next. This chapter will show you the way.

Maybe after getting this far, you're thinking, *I've got so much weight to lose,* or *I'm so heavy, I don't know where to begin.* Listen to me: Don't let your mind defeat you and sink your spirit. Take stock of how positive you feel right now. Whether you lost 3 pounds,

10 pounds, or even more, you've already started to see and feel a difference in your body. You look better, and that's always something that makes you feel good. You're trimmer. Your skin is glowing. You have the radiant look that only good nutrition and proper exercise can produce. You've slimmed down to a smaller dress or pant size, and your body feels great. Your entire outlook has changed. These are just the jump starts that most people, including you, need to stay the course. With the *6-Day Body Makeover*, your body is now programmed to lose weight and shed fat at a steady pace. If you are happy with your results after six days and want to lose even more weight, this chapter provides instructions and resources for what you must do now, in a step-by-step fashion.

The *6-Day Body Makeover* is designed as a short-term program, and you should not stay on it indefinitely (no more than 6 to 10 days). However, with the information in this chapter, you'll learn how to adjust the program to keep losing weight and live a lifestyle that keeps you toned and trim. If you don't yet have the body you want, don't worry. Maybe you're close, but realistically, it usually takes a little longer to achieve your dream body. The amount of time it takes to reach your goal weight depends on how much weight you have to lose in the first place. If you had 10 pounds to lose, you may have already achieved your goal. But if you had 20 or more, it will take longer.

Here's the good news, though: You can keep on going with an expanded, more liberal version of the *6-Day Body Makeover*. I will show you how to tweak and expand the program so that it will keep working, and your body will continue to lose weight. No matter how much weight you want to lose, you can drop every pound of your excess weight—and do it with lifelong results.

Remember to be patient with yourself. You've already made significant progress. Now you're armed with the knowledge you need to change your body. As long as you continue with the program, it will be just a matter of time before you will have that dream body.

The Next Step

Trust me on this: You *can* keep the body you've created, or are in the process of creating, by following the eight-step plan below. The meals in your *6-Day Body Makeover* custom eating plan were designed to recharge your body's metabolism so that you lost weight quickly. To keep that momentum going, you can begin to expand on those meal plans without sacrificing your shape or the new clothing size you're wearing.

Now that your body's metabolism is at the point that it burns off fat very quickly, you'll find that you can introduce extra carbohydrates, fruits, and other types of protein back into your eating program—foods you had to limit in order to rapidly lose weight. So from this point forward, you'll enjoy expanded food choices. For example, perhaps you'd like to eat a little more red meat than is currently on your plan, or enjoy a wider selection of fruits. Go ahead and do it. You'll often find that when your metabolism is so revved up, it will quickly burn through most foods without any problem.

The steps below are geared to help you lose more weight, or ease into maintaining the weight you just lost. Hopefully, you've begun to develop the habit of keeping an eye on your body. You've watched it change even in the last six days. So as you follow these guidelines, see how your body responds. If something isn't working, change it. You may need to cut back on choices such as eating red meat, or reducing your portions of certain carbohydrates. But whatever you implement, make sure that it involves five to six meals of wholesome, clean-burning fuel spread out over the day. Here's how to proceed.

Step 1: Expand Your Carbohydrate Choices

To maintain your six-day weight loss, or to continue losing additional pounds, the main dietary adjustment you need to make is to add extra servings of starchy carbohydrates and fruits back into your diet. As for greens and other vegetables, you can generally add as many of these foods back in as you like without affecting your metabolism.

How many servings should you add? A good rule of thumb for transitioning into further weight loss or into maintenance is to eat one additional serving of carbohydrate and one additional serving of fruit each day. For example, if your six-day eating plan called for one fruit, now you can eat two fruits. Similarly, if your six-day eating plan specified two servings of starchy carbohydrates, now you can enjoy three servings. The key is to not go overboard now that the six days are up. If you immediately return to your old ways of eating, you'll return to your old size in no time at all!

Here is an expanded list of carbohydrates and fruits from which you can plan your meals:

Starchy Carbohydrates

Barley

Jicama

Millet

Oat bran

Oatmeal

Potatoes

Rutabagas

Squash, winter

Sweet potatoes

Turnips/parsnips

Rice (brown rice, long-
grain rice, and wild rice
are best)

Rice noodles

Whole-grain hot cereals,
such as Cream of Rice or
Cream of Wheat

Fruits*

Apple

Banana

Cantaloupe and other
melons

Nectarine

Papaya

Peach

Pear

Pineapple

Plum

---

*I believe that it is best for optimum metabolic functioning if you choose fresh fruits. However, you can use frozen or canned fruits, as long as they are not packed in sugar or syrup. For canned fruits, look for those products packed in water or in their own juice.

Step 2: Expand Your Protein Choices

No longer are you limited to just egg whites, certain types of fish, and lean poultry. Feel free to expand your protein choices to include shellfish, fattier types of fish such as salmon or swordfish, lean red meat (even if it wasn't on your six-day plan), and lean cuts of pork.

Proteins

Crab

Beef, lean cuts

Lobster

Pork, lean chops

Pork, lean tenderloin

Salmon

Scallops

Shrimp

Swordfish

All varieties of fish

Step 3: Stay Consistent with Your Portion Sizes

This is very important: Stick to the same portion sizes you used while following the *6-Day Body Makeover*. These portions represent the precise amount of food your body can metabolize and use for fuel without being stored as fat. You've just spent six days learning how to manage your portion sizes. This period of time should help reinforce the healthy habit of portion management. Continue to weigh and measure your foods, or use the chart on page 45 as a guideline, to ensure that you're not eating more than your metabolism can process.

Step 4: Continue to Customize for Your Body Type

Select specific foods geared to your body type in order to keep your metabolism racing along at a good fat-burning pace. Thus, I want you to stick to the basic template of the customized eating plan you followed on the *6-Day Body Makeover*, but be sure to use the expanded food choices listed above, adding in extra servings of starchy carbohydrates and fruits. Here are some examples of how to customize for further weight loss and/or maintenance:

BODY TYPE A (ENDOMORPH)

- Enjoy a carbohydrate such as oatmeal for breakfast. Thus, a good breakfast for you would be scrambled egg whites and oatmeal.

- For your midmorning and midafternoon snacks, have a carbohydrate such as rice, a potato, or a sweet potato, rather than greens, with your protein.

- At lunch and dinner, vary your starchy carbohydrate choices by selecting from the expanded list above.

- At most meals, including snacks, vary your protein choices, using the list above as a guideline.

- If you opt for your PM snack, have some fresh fruit with your protein, instead of greens.

A typical meal on your plan would be: Herb-Crusted Fish (page 191; use a fish such as red snapper or flounder), roasted new potatoes, and a green salad. This certainly isn't what most people think of as diet food, but it is precisely the type of food your body needs to keep its metabolism running in high gear and help you lose weight!

BODY TYPE B (ENDO-MESO)

- Vary your fruit choices considerably at breakfast and for your PM snack.

- Substitute fruit for greens at your midmorning snack.

- Increase your carbohydrate intake by having a starchy carbohydrate such as a potato or rice for your midafternoon snack, rather than greens.

- Vary your protein and carbohydrate choices at lunch and dinner.

A typical meal on your plan would be: Chicken breast sautéed in wine and garlic, mashed potatoes, and steamed asparagus. As long as you continue eating natural, delicious foods like this, in the right amounts, you'll never go hungry, and your body will have what it needs to achieve an efficient metabolic rate.

BODY TYPE C (MESO-ENDO)

- Add a starchy carbohydrate such as oatmeal or a potato to your breakfast meal.

- Increase your carbohydrate intake by having a starchy carb such as a sweet potato or rice at your midmorning and midafternoon snacks, instead of greens.

- Use the expanded lists of carbohydrates, fruits, and protein to vary all your daily menu selections.

A typical meal on your plan would be: Steeped Chicken (page 199), stir-fried vegetables, and rice noodles. This is a great time to get creative with your meals. With a little bit of effort, you can create meals designed to work with your body chemistry that your entire family will enjoy. Continue to use appendix A for ideas on how to create mouthwatering meals that do not taste like diet food.

BODY TYPE D (ENDO-ECTO)

- When you followed your customized eating plan on the *6-Day Body Makeover,* your breakfast was pure protein. Now feel free to add a starchy carbohydrate such as oatmeal or oat bran at breakfast for more variety.

- For snacks, enjoy fruit with your protein, as a substitute for greens.

- Vary your menus as much as possible by selecting from the expanded food lists.

A typical meal on your plan would be: Grilled New York strip steak, Oven-Baked French Fries (page 209), and Grilled Vegetables (page 205). Remember that eating all the food on your plan is very important, because if you skip meals or skimp on portion sizes, the plan will not work.

BODY TYPE E (ECTO-ENDO)

- Start the day with a bigger breakfast that includes a hot whole-grain cereal such as Cream of Wheat and a serving of fruit (refer to the expanded lists above).

- Increase your starchy carbohydrate intake again at your midmorning snack by enjoying a carbohydrate such as winter squash or a potato, instead of greens.

- Vary your menus as much as possible by selecting from the expanded food lists of starchy carbohydrates, fruits, and proteins.

A typical meal on your plan would be: Roast pork tenderloin, mashed winter squash, and green beans. This is the type of meal you can eat for lunch or dinner. You can go ahead and increase the amount of greens and vegetables you eat at these meals if you like to fill up your plate.

Step 5: Continue to Water Your Body

Very important: You still must continue to drink 12 glasses of water (100 ounces) every day to ensure the steady burning of fat. Occasionally, it is permissible to have diet drinks, but do not include them as part of your daily fluid intake.

Step 6: Avoid Fat-Forming Foods

For additional, ongoing weight loss, be careful with certain foods that could slow or halt your progress altogether. These include:

- Oils: especially tropical, saturated types.
- Fats: especially animal fat, butter, and nuts.
- Dairy: Milk, sour cream, any kind of cheese, and ice cream.
- Fruits: Coconuts, dates, fruits canned or packaged in syrup or sugar (fruits canned in water or in their own juice are fine, as are frozen unsweetened fruits).
- Processed foods: breads, pastas, flour products, and deli meat.
- Liquids: sugared sodas, alcohol, milk, fruit and vegetable juices.
- Salt: This is a must, unless you have low blood pressure.

Step 7: Maintain Positive Eating Habits

Over the past six days, you began developing eating habits that will help you not only take off more weight, but also maintain that weight loss. These habits are ones you'll want to keep up. For example:

- Eating five to six times a day.
- Not eating in excess of what your body and metabolism can handle.
- Planning the week's meals ahead of time and preparing some foods in bulk for convenience.
- Eating foods that are as fresh and as wholesome as possible.

Step 8: Monitor and Review Your Weight Periodically

One of the habits of people who lose weight and keep it off is that they self-monitor, meaning they weigh themselves on a periodic basis to track weight fluctuations early so

Beyond the *6-Day Body Makeover*, you can enjoy occasional meals at restaurants. As long as you're careful, you can stay on your custom eating plan and still continue to shed pounds at a steady rate. More and more restaurants are now health-conscious and accommodating about preparing foods in a more nutritious way by adding low-calorie, low-fat, and low-sodium foods to their menus. Don't be shy about asking your server to have your food prepared with minimum fat, oil, or salt. It's better to eat something, even if it is not exactly like what's on your meal plan. Just be sure to choose and order wisely. For example, you can order:

- Sashimi
- Fish or chicken breast that is broiled or grilled
- Seafood en brochette, grilled, boiled, or steamed
- Lean beef that is grilled (eat a smaller portion; take the rest home)

- Vegetables en brochette, grilled, boiled, or steamed
- Plain baked potato
- Salad with lemon, vinegar, and/or herbs
- Fruit or fruit sorbet for dessert

that they can take action. If your weight starts to rise or your clothes feel tight again, this feedback can help you deal with it before it gets out of hand. You may have to become stricter with your eating plan or portion sizes, check your sodium intake, increase your exercise effort, or go back on the *6-Day Body Makeover*.

I'm not saying that you should go crazy over every pound you go up (because it could be temporary water weight), but I do want you to be aware of a steady or sudden gain in weight so that you can make further adjustments to your eating and exercise plans.

Staying Active

You've successfully completed the *6-Day Body Makeover,* and you're committed to keeping your weight off or going on to lose more. And you've hit the ground walking or jogging with long slow distance exercise. No doubt about it: You're on the right track to weight control. But well-made-over bodies aren't just fat-free—they're firm!

Take another look at yourself in the mirror. If despite the pounds and inches you've lost, you need some tone and definition here and there, it's time to start a serious weight-training program. This form of exercise, also called resistance training, is absolutely essential to successful weight loss and lifelong weight maintenance. In fact, it is one of the main tools used by people who have kept their weight off for years and years.

Weight training is important to weight control because it builds metabolically active muscle tissue. The more muscle there is on your body, the more efficient your metabolism is, since muscle burns calories, even at rest. This helps any surplus of fat melt off your body and is among the best ways to keep flab off. Unless you weight train, you can lose an average of ½ pound of muscle each year after the age of 25. But with resistance training, even muscle that is often lost to aging can be regained. When you do weight training or apply some sort of resistance to challenge your muscles, you actually break down muscle cells. Then with rest and proper nutrition, they heal, but become stronger and more shapely as they regenerate. Incorporating resistance training into your routine is a part of the deep-seated lifestyle change you must make to be successful at weight control.

To my women readers: You may be concerned that if you lift weights, you'll develop large, bulky muscles—and start looking like the Incredible Hulk. Nothing could be farther from the truth. You'll look incredible if you lift weights, but you certainly won't look like a hulk. Women simply do not have enough male hormones in their bodies to develop big muscles. What will happen is that by lifting weights or doing some other form of resistance training, you'll firm up and tone up in all the right places, and look sexier and more attractive than you have in years. All forms of resistance training have the power to radically transform your figure in ways you never dreamed possible. So no matter what your age, if you want to go from fat to firm in a relatively short time period, you must begin a resistance-training program.

Getting Started

Exercising your muscles against resistance involves the use of weights (barbells or dumbbells), weight-training machines that are designed for home or gym use, exercise bands, or even your own body. Here are some specifics:

- *Barbells and dumbbells* come in various poundages, lengths, and grips, and there are literally hundreds of exercises you can perform with them.

- *Weight machines.* Designed to work specific body parts, weight machines let you adjust the poundage according to the amount of resistance you want to use. They guide you through a specific range of motion—the full path of an exercise repetition, from beginning to end and back again.

- *Exercise bands* are tubes of flexible, stretchable rubber with handles on the ends for comfort and easy use. You can use bands to work almost any muscle group, including triceps, biceps, chest, back, shoulders, thighs, hamstrings, abdominals, and many more. Available in sporting goods stores and through the Internet, exercise bands typically come in several different levels of difficulty, which is determined by the elasticity of the band and marked by its color. Some come with door anchors and clips so that you can attach the bands to doorways in order to perform the exercises.

- *Your own body weight.* Many exercises can be performed using your own body weight as resistance. Some familiar examples include push-ups, pull-ups, abdominal crunches, and knee bends.

The first decision you'll want to make regarding resistance training is whether to work out at home or at a gym. Working out at home is convenient, since you can exercise when your schedule permits it without worrying about driving back and forth from a gym. All you need to equip yourself for working out at home is a set of dumbbells and barbells and/or exercise bands. You can also perform exercises that use your own body weight as resistance.

On the other hand, you may prefer to work out at a gym, where there is usually a wide variety of equipment and often more exercise options. When choosing a gym, make sure it's convenient, affordable, and well staffed with qualified people such as personal trainers who can show you the ropes, particularly if you're a newcomer to resistance training and need individualized instruction. Of course, you don't need a personal trainer forever—just long enough for someone to show you the dos and don'ts and help you sculpt your body to your full satisfaction. Trainers are a great resource when you're first getting started and if you need the continual motivation they can provide.

Whether you work out at home or at a gym, here are some important guidelines to observe as you prepare to start a resistance-training program:

- Perform resistance training twice or three times a week, allowing two to three days between workouts in order to let your muscles recuperate or adapt so that they can change shape. It's best to schedule your individual workouts so that they occur on the same day of every week. That way, you're always assured of getting enough rest in between each session. For instance, if you schedule your first routine on Monday and your second routine on Wednesday, stick to that schedule every week. Then each muscle has a full week in which to adapt and change.

- When setting up your exercise routine, include at least one exercise for each of your major body parts: thighs, chest, back, shoulders, arms, abdominals, and calves.

- Concentrate on those muscles that need extra shape, tone, and definition. If your legs are already fairly muscular, for example, then you don't have to train them as hard or as often. But if your abs are flab, then that's an area you'd want to focus on with more intensified exercise. That's the beauty of resistance training: You can add or subtract inches simply by the exercise choices you make.

- Warm up first with approximately 10 minutes of light aerobic activity: walking on a treadmill, riding a stationary bicycle, walking around a track, or simply running in place. These activities slightly elevate your muscle temperature to prepare your body for the exercises.

- When you first try an exercise, use a light resistance—one that you can comfortably lift for about 12 repetitions—to get a feel for the movement. The last two to three repetitions should feel more difficult and require extra effort.

- On the lifting and lowering portion of exercises, control the resistance smoothly and slowly, without letting momentum take over. Don't jerk through the exercise—this can endanger your joints.

- Always use proper form during an exercise. If you need to contort your body in some way to lift a certain poundage or resistance, then that resistance is too heavy for you and you risk injury to a muscle or joint.

- Perform two to three sets of each exercise. (A *set* is a series of repetitions.) Rest for 30 seconds to one minute between exercise sets.

- Challenge your muscles each time you work out. Generally, when you can perform more than 15 repetitions without much effort, it's time to increase the weight or the resistance. Pushing a little harder against resistance builds strength and develops lean, beautiful muscle.

The important issue is that you add some form of resistance training to your overall health and fitness routine. It will help you reshape your body. It will keep you looking and feeling youthful. And it is one of the best ways to keep lost weight off your body, forever.

Further Options: The *6-Week Body Makeover*

Depending on what shape your body is currently in, a true body makeover may take longer than six days and may involve special exercises to sculpt your body. As you've found, six days of customized eating and long slow distance exercise takes enough fat off in the right places to make it easy to fit into a dress or pants that are a whole size smaller. But to truly make over your entire body, you need more time—though not a lot more time. Depending on what you want to achieve, as well as your starting weight and shape, you can make over your entire body in as little as six weeks, using the guidelines in this chapter. However, you may want to consider graduating to the *6-Week Body Makeover*. This is a packaged system of diet and exercise tools that provides detailed, customized approaches and methods similar to those of the six-day program, but is more liberal and flexible in its food choices.

As part of my *6-Week Body Makeover*, I developed the Precision Body Sculpting System to target, reshape, and make over your problem areas. Using exercise bands, this routine requires only 15 to 18 minutes of exercise, just twice a week, to firm and tone your hips, thighs, and buns; get tight, sexy abs; and even lift your bosom and improve your posture. All in as little as six weeks!

With your new knowledge of how food influences your own individual body chemistry, and exercise influences your body type, you now have the secret to controlling your weight for the rest of your life. The decision of whether to eat according to your Body Type Blueprint or not will always be yours, and the *6-Week Body Makeover* program may provide additional tools and information to help you do so. With the *6-Week Body Makeover*, for example, you can pick exactly what you want your body to look like, then make it over to your exact specifications. You get to design (down to the last detail), then create, the ideal body. For women, if you want to slim your waist, create firm, shapely arms, and enjoy defined, sexy legs, you can do exactly that. For guys, if you want to sculpt washboard abs, broad shoulders, a V-shaped back, and strong, well-defined arms, that's precisely what you can do. The *6-Week Body Makeover* is totally customized to you and is designed to give you *exactly* the body you want.

If you would like more information on how you can get started on the *6-Week Body Makeover*, please refer to appendix C. Here are the photos and stories of some inspirational women who will provide you with the incentive to continue with your weight-loss program.

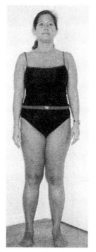

Before

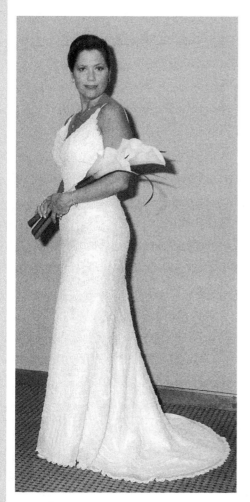

After

Nancy B.

After trying numerous diets, Nancy lost 40 pounds on my *6-Week Body Make-over*—more weight than she'd ever lost in her life. What's more, she has successfully used the *6-Day Body Makeover* several times. "It is amazing and really works!" she says. "I use it when I feel like I've added a few pounds and want to get them off quickly, or when I'm on a plateau it seems to shake things up and start the weight loss again. I've lost anywhere from 4 to 6 pounds in six days and easily an inch or more on my waist. It is just enough to feel good in the pants that were once just too snug." In addition, Nancy used the *6-Day Body Makeover* to get in shape for the most important day of her life—her wedding.

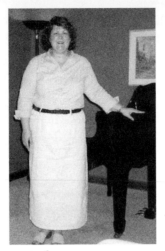

Before

Sally P.

Sally's story is typical of many dieters: She gained weight with the birth of each of her eight children, and tried to lose it with one diet after another but without any lasting success. Eventually, Sally dieted her way up to 217 pounds. Frustrated, she tried my *6-Week Body Makeover*. It worked for her. She is now a size 8. Part of her strategy involved using the *6-Day Body Makeover*. One summer she used it to get from a size 18 to a size 16, and lost 9 pounds in the process. Today, Sally uses the *6-Day Body Makeover* whenever her weight creeps up a bit—and to maintain her lovely size 8.

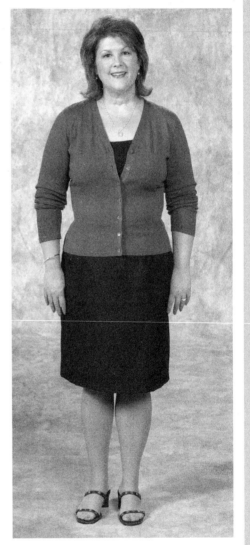

After

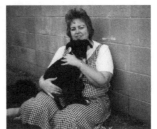

Before

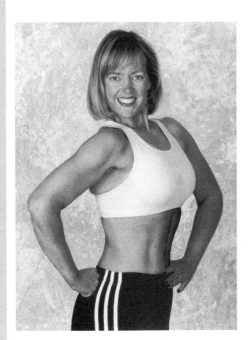

After

Dolores T.

Weight problems plagued Dolores all her life—and so did yo-yo dieting. The weight always returned and then some. In September 1998, she tried my *6-Week Body Makeover,* eventually losing 92 pounds and 84 inches. Equally as impressive: Dolores has kept that weight off for six years. Like so many of my makeover clients, Dolores has used the *6-Day Body Makeover* on many occasions, particularly vacations. "To get ready for a trip to Jamaica with my husband, I went on the *6-Day Body Makeover,*" she says. "I had never ever worn a two-piece bathing suit in my life, but I did after that experience! I easily lost a size that week."

When to Use the *6-Day Body Makeover* Again

Even though you may choose to continue with the step-by-step plan above, or with the *6-Week Body Makeover,* never forget that you always have the *6-Day Body Makeover* to use as a tool to manage your weight, stay at your desired clothing size, and maintain the body of your dreams. You just never know when the *6-Day Body Makeover* will come in handy!

Here's a case in point: Dolores, whose photo is featured on page 179, had a weight problem all her life, including being an overweight child all through school. She was the typical yo-yo dieter who went on and off many different diet programs, without any sustainable success. "When I would manage to lose some weight, it *always* came back," she told me. "Oftentimes with more added on for good measure."

Dolores began my *6-Week Body Makeover* in September 1998, weighing 237 pounds and wearing a size 22. She successfully lost an incredible 92 pounds and 84 inches and has kept the weight off for more than six years. Dolores describes it like this: "Maintaining my lost weight was always a major problem, but not this time! My life has changed in so many ways and so many new doors have opened up for me. I so loved the feeling of being fit and healthy for the first time in my life that I went on to become a personal fitness trainer and a certified sports nutrition specialist. I have favorably influenced so many family members, friends, and co-workers who wanted to know how I did it and as a result have turned them onto this fabulous program. My own brother-in-law lost an amazing 114 pounds!"

Just recently, Dolores was set to take a vacation with her husband to Jamaica, and she wanted to lose a few pounds in order to get back down to her goal weight of 145 pounds. So she went on the *6-Day Body Makeover.* Dolores easily lost one whole size that week, but the best news of all was that she was able to look terrific in a two-piece bathing suit. Now Dolores uses the *6-Day Body Makeover* routinely when she wants to look her absolute best.

I hope that for you, as for my many clients, concluding the *6-Day Body Makeover* has signaled not an end, but a new beginning, with a trimmer, better-looking, sexier body. You've started a whole new way of being in this world—healthier, more energetic, more beautiful. You no longer have to starve to try to get down to size. You no longer have to settle for diet food that's devoid of natural nutrients, or grueling exercise that takes up time without taking off pounds. Instead, you've gained a new perspective on what it's like to look and feel your best.

Maybe like so many people I've worked with, you feel so much better about yourself in general. You feel really great every day—a fitness of mind and body that communicates to everyone your newfound self-confidence, your endless supply of energy, and your radiant health. It is this sense of confidence that will keep you going for the long term, and cement your desire to stay in fabulous shape.

I want to tell you again from the bottom of my heart: Congratulations! You've proved you can succeed—and with less toil and trouble than you've ever before experienced! You look great. Show off the new you to the world. You deserve the best. Now go out there and live it.

The 6-Day Body Makeover *Recipes*

To make the next six days as interesting and enjoyable as possible, use the following recipes, which have been created expressly for all of my makeover programs. These recipes are designed to add flavor and variety to the way you prepare and eat your food. Although your food on the *6-Day Body Makeover* must be measured and weighed, you do have a lot of leeway in how you season it. The only rule carved in stone is that you must not use any salt, oil, dairy products, or sugar in preparing your meals. If you see a recipe for fish or poultry that looks appealing, go for it. Do whatever you need to do, within the parameters and guidelines of this program, to keep your food tasting delicious.

As a handy reference, you'll find a code with each recipe that tells you which body type and meal the recipe matches. That way, you can select only the recipes that correspond to your custom eating plan.

Marinades

Marinating serves two purposes: It tenderizes meat, and it adds flavor. So if you can, take the time to marinate fish or poultry. Fish usually does not require a long marinating time—usually only half an hour prior to cooking. For best results, chicken and turkey usually require several hours to marinate. Always refrigerate fish or meat when marinating for more than a few minutes.

CUBAN LIME MARINADE

> 3 cloves garlic
> 2 tsp. ground cumin
> ½ cup fresh lime juice
> 1 tbsp. chopped fresh oregano
> ½ tsp. ground black pepper

Mash the garlic with a mortar and pestle, or press it through a garlic press to make it into a smooth paste. Add the cumin, lime juice, oregano, and pepper. Use this mixture to marinate chicken or turkey breast in the refrigerator for several hours prior to cooking. This recipe makes enough marinade for 2 servings.

Compatible with Body Types:
> Breakfast: **A, B, C, D, E**
> Midmorning Snack: **A, B, C, D, E**
> Lunch: **A, B, C, D, E**
> Midafternoon Snack: **A, B, C, D**
> Dinner: **A, B, C, D, E**
> PM Snack: **A, D, E**

INDIAN MARINADE

> 1½ tbsp. minced fresh gingerroot
> 4 cloves garlic, minced or pressed
> 2 jalapeño peppers, chopped

½ cup lemon juice

2 bay leaves

2 tsp. paprika

1 tsp. ground turmeric

½ tsp. ground cardamom

1½ tsp. ground ginger

½ tsp. ground cinnamon

½ tsp. freshly ground black pepper

Combine the fresh ginger, garlic, and peppers in a bowl. Add the lemon juice, bay leaves, and remaining spices. Use the mixture to marinate chicken or turkey breast in the refrigerator for several hours prior to cooking. This recipe makes enough marinade for 2 servings; you may double it for additional servings.

Compatible with Body Types:

Breakfast: **A, B, C, D, E**

Midmorning Snack: **A, B, C, D, E**

Lunch: **A, B, C, D, E**

Midafternoon Snack: **A, B, C, D**

Dinner: **A, B, C, D, E**

PM Snack: **A, D, E**

THAI MARINADE

¼ cup fresh parsley, minced

¼ cup lemon juice

½ tsp. grated fresh gingerroot

¼ cup lime juice

1 tsp. red pepper flakes

3 cloves garlic, minced or pressed

Combine all ingredients. Use this mixture to marinate fish, chicken, or turkey breast in the refrigerator for several hours prior to cooking. This recipe makes enough marinade for 2 servings and can be doubled for more servings.

Compatible with Body Types:
    Breakfast: **A, B, C, D, E**
    Midmorning Snack: **A, B, C, D, E**
    Lunch: **A, B, C, D, E**
    Midafternoon Snack: **A, B, C, D**
    Dinner: **A, B, C, D, E**
    PM Snack: **A, D, E**

Fish

Fish is an excellent weight-control food since it metabolizes quickly and thus facilitates rapid weight loss. If you don't like fish, I recommend that you at least give it a shot by trying new and creative ways to prepare it. You might enjoy milder varieties of fish such as red snapper or orange roughy seasoned well with lemon juice and herbs and spices, or any of the recipes listed below.

GRILLED RED SNAPPER WITH FENNEL

    1 lb. red snapper
    ½ cup lemon or lime juice
    1 tsp. freshly grated gingerroot
    1 tsp. freshly grated pepper
    Scallions, cut into 1-inch pieces
    ½ fennel bulb, trimmed and cut into 1-inch pieces

In a shallow baking dish, place the fish in a single layer. Combine the lemon juice with the gingerroot and pepper. Pour over the fish and marinate in the refrigerator for 2 hours. Remove the fish from the marinade. Scatter the scallions and fennel over the fish, then wrap it securely in aluminum foil and grill (or bake at 350 degrees) for 20 to 30 minutes, or until it flakes easily with a fork. Serve immediately. You may substitute any type of fish for snapper. Makes 3 to 4 servings.

Compatible with Body Types:
>Breakfast: N/A
>Midmorning Snack: **A**
>Lunch: **A**
>Midafternoon Snack: **A, B, C**
>Dinner: **A**
>PM Snack: **D**

BAKED FISH FILLETS WITH MUSHROOMS AND TOMATOES

>1 onion, chopped
>3 stalks celery, chopped
>1 cup mushrooms, sliced
>2 tbsp. fresh dill or rosemary
>1 lb. haddock or cod fillets
>Lemon juice, fresh
>Freshly grated pepper
>4 tomatoes, sliced

Preheat the oven to 375 degrees. Sauté the onion, celery, and mushrooms briefly in a few tablespoons of water. Add the dill or rosemary. Arrange the vegetables in a baking dish. Place the fish on top. Sprinkle with fresh lemon juice and some freshly grated pepper, then cover the fish with sliced toma-toes. Bake, uncovered, for 35 to 40 minutes. If necessary, add a slight amount of water to prevent the fish from drying while it bakes. You can substitute chicken or turkey for the fish. Makes 3 to 4 servings.

Compatible with Body Types:
   Breakfast: N/A
   Midmorning Snack: **A, B, C, D, E**
   Lunch: **A, B, C, D, E**
   Midafternoon Snack: **A, B, C, D**
   Dinner: **A, B, C, D, E**
   PM Snack: **A, D**

GRILLED TUNA STEAK

   4 tuna steaks
   Juice of 2 limes
   1 tbsp. marjoram
   2 cloves garlic, pressed or minced

Marinate the tuna steaks in the lime juice with the marjoram and garlic. Grill about 10 minutes on each side, basting with marinade. Makes 4 servings.

Compatible with Body Types:
   Breakfast: N/A
   Midmorning Snack: **A**
   Lunch: **A**
   Midafternoon Snack: **A, B, C**
   Dinner: **A**
   PM Snack: **D**

FISH AND VEGETABLE KEBABS

1 lb. firm-textured fish such as halibut or shark

1 large red onion, sliced

2 large green or yellow peppers, seeded and cut into 1-inch pieces

2 small zucchini, sliced

8 to 10 large mushrooms

MARINADE:

½ cup lemon juice

¼ teaspoon pepper

2 tbsp. minced fresh gingerroot

1 clove garlic, minced or pressed

Combine the marinade ingredients. Cut the fish into 1-inch pieces and place in the marinade. Cover and refrigerate for 2 to 3 hours. Remove the fish from the marinade. Add the onion, peppers, zucchini, and mushrooms to the marinade to coat. Place the fish and vegetables on skewers. Grill—turning carefully to cook on all sides—for approximately 10 minutes. The kebabs are done when the fish flakes when touched with a fork. If you prepare 4 kebabs, each one will have about 4 ounces of fish on it. If you make 8, each will contain about 3 ounces of fish. Plan your portion according to the amount of protein you are allotted on your particular diet. You can also substitute chicken breast for fish.

Compatible with Body Types:

Breakfast: N/A

Midmorning Snack: **A, D, E**

Lunch: **A, B, C, D, E**

Midafternoon Snack: **A, B, C, D**

Dinner: **A, B, C, D, E**

PM Snack: **A, D**

STEAM-POACHED FISH FILLETS

1 lb. halibut or red snapper fillets

6 sprigs parsley

1 bay leaf

2 cloves garlic, minced or pressed

10 to 12 mushrooms, whole or sliced

1 onion, sliced thin

5 to 6 tomatoes, sliced

1 green pepper, seeded and sliced

Cut the fish into 2-ounce slices and place on a piece of foil large enough to cover the fish and vegetables. Top the fish with the parsley, bay leaf, and garlic. Cover with vegetables. Wrap securely with the foil, being sure to seal the edges. You can steam these in a steamer on the stove or place the foil packet on top of a rack that is placed in an ovenproof baking dish filled with 2 inches of boiling water. Poach for about 12 to 15 minutes. Test the fish for doneness by cutting it with a knife; it's done when it's no longer translucent. Remove the bay leaf prior to serving. Makes 3 to 4 servings.

Compatible with Body Types:
    Breakfast: N/A
    Midmorning Snack: **A**
    Lunch: **A**
    Midafternoon Snack: **A, B, C**
    Dinner: **A**
    PM Snack: **D**

HERB-CRUSTED FISH

Juice of 1 lemon
1 clove garlic, minced
4 to 6 cups fresh cilantro, chopped
2 lbs. flounder fillets

Preheat the oven to 350 degrees. Mix the lemon juice and garlic in one bowl. Place the cilantro in a separate bowl. Dip each fillet in the lemon juice, then dredge in the cilantro. Place in a baking dish and pour the remaining juice around the fillets.

Bake for 20 to 30 minutes or until the fish is fully cooked, basting periodically. The fish is done when it flakes easily with a fork. Makes 6 to 8 servings.

Compatible with Body Types:
Breakfast: N/A
Midmorning Snack: **A**
Lunch: **A**
Midafternoon Snack: **A, B, C**
Dinner: **A**
PM Snack: **D**

CEVICHE SALAD

1 lb. cooked sea bass fillet, cut into ½-inch cubes
Juice of 3 limes
1 medium red onion, thinly sliced
4 tomatoes, diced
1 green pepper, seeded and chopped
¼ cup fresh cilantro, chopped
½ tsp. freshly ground black pepper
2 cloves garlic, minced

Place the fish in a ceramic or glass bowl and combine with the lime juice. Add the remaining ingredients and stir carefully. Refrigerate for 2 to 3 hours. Serve cold. Makes 3 to 4 servings.

Compatible with Body Types:
  Breakfast: N/A
  Midmorning Snack: **A**
  Lunch: **A**
  Midafternoon Snack: **A, B, C**
  Dinner: **A**
  PM Snack: **D**

Poultry

When preparing chicken or turkey, select breast meat only. The portions below are based on using boneless, skinless chicken or turkey breasts. Never cook poultry with the skin on, since it is so full of fat. An average chicken breast is 4 ounces, so a 2-ounce serving is about one-half of a chicken breast. Nonetheless, weigh your portions so that you know exactly how much you're eating.

TURKEY SAUSAGE PATTIES

  1 lb. lean ground turkey breast
  ½ tsp. cumin
  ½ tsp. cayenne pepper
  ½ tsp. garlic powder
  1 tsp. coriander
  ¼ tsp. freshly ground black pepper
  1 tsp. paprika

½ tsp. oregano

½ tsp. basil

½ cup chicken broth, sodium- and fat-free

Combine the turkey and dry spices in a large bowl. Mix together thoroughly. Add the chicken broth, mixing well. Let stand for 15 to 20 minutes.

Form the turkey into 8 patties, approximately ¾ inch thick. Cook the patties in a nonstick skillet over medium heat for 7 to 8 minutes on each side or until thoroughly cooked. Makes four servings.

Compatible with Body Types:
Breakfast: **A, B, C, D, E**
Midmorning Snack: **B, C**
Lunch: N/A
Midafternoon Snack: N/A
Dinner: N/A
PM Snack: N/A

ORANGE AND GARLIC CHICKEN

Juice of 1 orange

1 tbsp. grated orange peel

2 cloves garlic, minced or pressed

1 tsp. chopped fresh rosemary

4 boneless skinless chicken breasts

½ tsp. pepper

2 tsp. paprika

Combine the juice of the orange with the orange peel, garlic, rosemary, and chicken. Marinate for 3 to 4 hours. Sprinkle the chicken with the pepper and paprika. Grill, boil, or sauté for 5 to 6 minutes on each side or until done. The chicken is done when it is no longer pink inside. Makes 4 servings.

Compatible with Body Types:
    Breakfast: N/A
    Midmorning Snack: **D, E**
    Lunch: **B, C, D, E**
    Midafternoon Snack: **D**
    Dinner: **B, C, D, E**
    PM Snack: **A, E**

ROAST CHICKEN WITH VEGETABLES

4 boneless skinless chicken breasts
4 to 5 tomatoes, chopped
1 cup sliced mushrooms
1 cup okra, sliced or left whole
1 small onion, chopped
2 tbsp. tomato sauce, sodium-free
2 to 3 cloves garlic
Oregano
Rosemary, fresh or dried
Pepper

Preheat the oven to 350 degrees. Place the chicken breasts in a nonstick baking pan. Place the tomatoes, mushrooms, okra, and onion with the chicken. Dilute the tomato sauce with 1 cup of water. Add the garlic and oregano and mix well. Pour over the chicken and vegetables. If the sauce is too thick, add a little water. Make sure the vegetables are well covered with the sauce so that they don't dry out. Sprinkle the rosemary over the mixture, adding pepper to taste. Cover with foil and bake for 30 to 40 minutes, or until the chicken is done. Makes 4 servings.

Compatible with Body Types:

Breakfast: N/A

Midmorning Snack: **D, E**

Lunch: **B, C, D, E**

Midafternoon Snack: **D**

Dinner: **B, C, D, E**

PM Snack: **A**

STUFFED PEPPERS

4 cups cooked rice

½ tsp. paprika

½ tsp. rosemary

½ tsp. dried oregano

½ tsp. dried basil

1 onion

2 cups sliced mushrooms

1 lb. ground turkey breast or ground chicken breast

2 to 3 cloves garlic

2 tbsp. tomato paste, sodium-free

8 green peppers

Preheat the oven to 350 degrees. In a small bowl, combine the cooked rice with the herbs. In a large nonstick skillet, sauté the onion and mushrooms. Add the ground poultry and garlic and cook until the meat is fully browned. Drain off any water and fat. Combine the poultry with the cooked rice and herbs. Dilute the tomato paste with water and stir into the rice-and-poultry mixture.

Slice the tops off the peppers. Core and remove the seeds, but save the tops. Steam the peppers for 7 to 8 minutes.

Spoon the rice mixture into the peppers and place on a nonstick baking dish. Cover the peppers with their tops. Any additional mixture can be placed around peppers. Cover the baking dish with foil. Bake for about an hour. Each pepper contains approximately ½ cup of rice and about 2 ounces of poultry.

Compatible with Body Types:
    Breakfast: N/A
    Midmorning Snack: N/A
    Lunch: **B, C, D, E**
    Midafternoon Snack: N/A
    Dinner: **B, C, D, E**
    PM Snack: N/A

CHICKEN AND ASPARAGUS STIR-FRY

    4 boneless skinless chicken breasts
    2 cloves garlic, minced or pressed
    1 tbsp. minced fresh gingerroot
    ½ lb. mushrooms, thinly sliced
    8 green onions, cut into 1-inch slices
    1 lb. asparagus, ends cut off and cut into 1-inch pieces

Heat a nonstick pan or wok. Add the chicken, garlic, and ginger and stir-fry until the chicken is done (when the center is no longer pink)—about 5 to 8 minutes. Remove the chicken. Add the mushrooms, onions, and asparagus and stir-fry for 1 to 2 minutes. Add the chicken, stirring for about 1 minute. Makes 4 servings.

Compatible with Body Types:
    Breakfast: N/A
    Midmorning Snack: **D, E**
    Lunch: **B, C, D, E**
    Midafternoon Snack: **D**
    Dinner: **B, C, D, E**
    PM Snack: **A**

LEMON OREGANO CHICKEN

4 boneless skinless chicken breasts
1 clove garlic, minced or pressed
1 tsp. grated lemon peel
½ tsp. freshly grated black pepper
1 tbsp. chopped fresh oregano
Juice of 1 lemon

Rub the chicken with the garlic and grated lemon peel. Sprinkle with the pepper. Grill or sauté until done. Just before the chicken is fully cooked, add the oregano. When the chicken is done, add the lemon juice. Makes 4 servings.

Compatible with Body Types:
    Breakfast: N/A
    Midmorning Snack: **D, E**
    Lunch: **B, C, D, E**
    Midafternoon Snack: **D**
    Dinner: **B, C, D, E**
    PM Snack: **A, E**

POACHED CHICKEN

4 boneless skinless chicken breasts (or fish fillets)
1 cup rice vinegar or herb-flavored vinegar
1 tbsp. minced fresh gingerroot
1 cup water
3 cloves garlic, minced or pressed
1 tbsp. minced orange rind

Place all the ingredients in a shallow pan and bring the liquid to a boil. Cover and simmer over low heat for about 20 to 25 minutes. Makes 4 servings.

Compatible with Body Types:
    Breakfast: N/A
    Midmorning Snack: **D, E**
    Lunch: **B, C, D, E**
    Midafternoon Snack: **D**
    Dinner: **B, C, D, E**
    PM Snack: **A, E**

SPICY CHICKEN

    4 boneless skinless chicken breasts
    3 cloves garlic, minced or pressed
    1 tsp. turmeric
    5 whole cloves
    ½ tsp. chili powder
    3 large onions, chopped
    1 tsp. minced fresh gingerroot
    2 tsp. cardamom
    1 cinnamon stick or ½ tsp. ground cinnamon

In a nonstick skillet, heat the chicken pieces and cook (turning often) for 10 minutes or until done. Remove the chicken. Add the remaining ingredients, cover, and cook over low heat for about 15 minutes, stirring occasionally; be careful not to burn the onions. Return the chicken pieces to the pan; cover and simmer over low heat, stirring occasionally, for 5 to 10 minutes. Makes 4 servings.

Compatible with Body Types:
    Breakfast: N/A
    Midmorning Snack: **D, E**
    Lunch: **B, C, D, E**
    Midafternoon Snack: **D**

Dinner: **B, C, D, E**

PM Snack: **A, E**

STEEPED CHICKEN

Steeping is a Chinese cooking method that can be adapted to produce low-fat, yet very tender and succulent chicken. Poultry is cooked in a tightly covered pot of very hot liquid without using any direct heat from the stove. The meat steeps gently in the remaining heat and, when served, is very smooth-textured and tasty. Flavoring the liquid with lemon, lime, or herbs also lends flavor to the meat.

> 4 boneless skinless chicken breasts
> 1 clove garlic, minced or pressed
> Various herbs (rosemary, oregano, basil, and so forth)
> 3 slices lemon
> 1 sprig fresh parsley

Place the chicken in a saucepan, adding enough water to cover it by about 2 inches. Remove the chicken. Add the remaining ingredients. Bring the water to a rolling boil. Remove from the heat and add the chicken immediately. Cover the pan tightly and let the chicken steep for 20 minutes. Do not uncover until the time is up. The chicken is done when the center is no longer pink.

Save the water for sautéing vegetables, cooking rice, or stir-frying. It will keep in your refrigerator for several days. You can also freeze it for use later. Makes 4 servings.

Compatible with Body Types:
>   Breakfast: N/A
>   Midmorning Snack: **D, E**
>   Lunch: **B, C, D, E**

Midafternoon Snack: **D**
Dinner: **B, C, D, E**
PM Snack: **A, E**

JAMAICAN CHICKEN

½ cup chopped green onions
2 tbsp. minced fresh gingerroot
1 bay leaf
1 tsp. coriander
½ tsp. ground allspice
½ cup lime juice
3 tbsp. fresh thyme
1 habanero chile pepper
1 tsp. freshly ground pepper
½ tsp. ground nutmeg
4 boneless skinless chicken breasts

Combine all the ingredients except the chicken, mixing well to blend. Coat the chicken with the spice mixture and marinate for several hours in the refrigerator. Grill the chicken on an outdoor or indoor grill (or broil) for 4 to 6 minutes on each side. Makes 4 servings.

Compatible with Body Types:
Breakfast: N/A
Midmorning Snack: **D, E**
Lunch: **B, C, D, E**
Midafternoon Snack: **D**
Dinner: **B, C, D, E**
PM Snack: **A, E**

FIVE-ALARM CHILI

1 lb. ground chicken or turkey

1 onion, chopped

1 clove garlic, minced

1 green pepper, seeded and chopped

1 14-oz. can pinto beans, drained and washed (to reduce sodium)

1 tsp. oregano

½ tsp. cumin

½ tsp. freshly ground black pepper

½ tsp. cayenne pepper

28 oz. canned diced tomatoes (sodium-free)

Brown the meat in a nonstick Dutch oven or large pot along with the onion, garlic, and green pepper over medium heat until the meat is fully cooked. Drain off any excess oil. Add the beans and spices. Stir together for 1 minute. Add the tomatoes and bring to a boil. Lower the heat and simmer on low for 10 to 15 minutes, stirring occasionally. Makes 4 servings.

Compatible with Body Types:

Breakfast: N/A

Midmorning Snack: N/A

Lunch: **E**

Midafternoon Snack: N/A

Dinner: **E**

PM Snack: N/A

CLASSIC MEAT LOAF

2 lbs. lean ground chicken or turkey
1 cup chopped onion
½ cup diced celery
1 clove garlic, minced
½ tsp. oregano
½ tsp. thyme
½ tsp. freshly ground black pepper
¼ cup chopped fresh parsley
1 cup rice, cooked
2 egg whites
1¼ cups tomato sauce, sodium-free, divided

Preheat the oven to 350 degrees. In a large bowl, mix the ground poultry, onion, celery, and garlic. Mix all the spices together, then add them to the poultry and blend well.

One at a time, add the rice, the egg whites, and 1 cup of the tomato sauce to the poultry mixture and blend thoroughly. Form the mixture into an oval-shaped loaf and place in the center of a nonstick loaf pan. Spread the remaining ¼ cup of tomato sauce over the top of the loaf.

Bake, uncovered, for 1¼ hours. Let sit for 5 minutes before serving. Makes 6 to 8 servings.

Compatible with Body Types:
Breakfast: N/A
Midmorning Snack: N/A
Lunch: **B, C, D, E**
Midafternoon Snack: N/A
Dinner: **B, C, D, E**
PM Snack: N/A

Vegetables, Side Dishes, and Salads

SALSA

> 5 large ripe tomatoes, diced
> 2 to 3 jalapeño peppers, chopped
> 1 serrano chile pepper, chopped
> ¼ cup fresh cilantro, chopped
> ½ tsp. black pepper
> 1 cup chopped white onion
> 4 green onions, chopped (*optional*)
> ½ cup fresh lime or lemon juice
> 2 cloves garlic, pressed or chopped

Combine all the ingredients in a bowl. Take about a quarter of the mixture and process in a blender until liquefied. Mix back in with the remaining ingredients. If you like your salsa very hot, add a fourth jalapeño pepper (chopped) to the mixture. On the other hand, if you like milder salsa, omit the jalapeño peppers altogether, or use just one. This salsa will keep in the refrigerator for up to 3 days. To store longer, you may freeze it. This salsa is delicious when served over baked or broiled fish or chicken, mixed with cooked rice, or used as a dip for fresh vegetables.

Compatible with Body Types:
Breakfast: **A, B, C, D, E**
Midmorning Snack: **A, B, C, D, E**
Lunch: **A, B, C, D, E**
Midafternoon Snack: **A, B, C, D, E**
Dinner: **A, B, C, D, E**
PM Snack: **A, D**

VEGETABLE BROTH

If you are ambitious and want to make your own broth to sauté vegetables, fish, or chicken, this recipe is a good one to have on hand. You can also use this broth for cooking rice.

2 leeks
1 onion
1 cup mushrooms
1 bay leaf
½ cup fresh parsley
Freshly ground pepper
3 ribs celery
2 tomatoes
4 cloves garlic
½ cup fresh cilantro

Chop all the ingredients very finely and combine in a stockpot with 1½ to 2 quarts of water. Bring the water to a boil. Turn the heat down and simmer for 40 to 45 minutes. Strain out the vegetables and bay leaf and store the broth, tightly covered, in the refrigerator for up to 1 week.

Compatible with Body Types:
Breakfast: **A, B, C, D, E**
Midmorning Snack: **A, B, C, D, E**
Lunch: **A, B, C, D, E**
Midafternoon Snack: **A, B, C, D, E**
Dinner: **A, B, C, D, E**
PM Snack: **A, B, C, D, E**

GRILLED VEGETABLES

½ cup lemon juice
1 tbsp. oregano
3 cloves garlic, pressed
2 lbs. assorted fresh vegetables of your choice (such as eggplant, summer squash, zucchini, mushrooms, and onions)

Combine the lemon juice, oregano, and garlic. Slice the eggplant into ½-inch rounds. If the squash is too large, cut it in half lengthwise; if it is small, cut it into ½-inch pieces. Cut the peppers into large chunks; cut the onions into wedges or large rounds. Prepare any other vegetables you've chosen by cutting them into similar-sized chunks. Toss the vegetables in the lemon-and-herb mixture to coat, then place them in a single layer on a grill, or skewer like shish kebabs. Cover and grill for 10 to 20 minutes or until tender. Turn once and baste with any remaining lemon-herb mixture. Makes 4 servings.

Compatible with Body Types:
Breakfast: N/A
Midmorning Snack: **A, B, C, D, E**
Lunch: **A, B, C, D, E**
Midafternoon Snack: **A, B, C, D**
Dinner: **A, B, C, D, E**
PM Snack: **A, D**

RATATOUILLE

1 eggplant

3 cloves garlic, minced or pressed

1 green pepper

3 zucchini, sliced

1 tbsp. chopped fresh basil

1 tbsp. chopped fresh dill

Black pepper

1 onion

1 red pepper

1 yellow pepper

5 tomatoes, quartered

1 tbsp. chopped fresh tarragon

Cut the eggplant in half. Place it cut-side down on a nonstick cookie sheet and bake at 375 degrees for 40 to 45 minutes or until tender when pierced with a knife. Let the eggplant cool, then chop it into cubes. In a large non-stick pan, simmer the eggplant with the remaining ingredients for about 10 minutes, then serve warm or at room temperature. Makes 4 servings.

Compatible with Body Types:

Breakfast: N/A

Midmorning Snack: **A, B, C, D, E**

Lunch: **A, B, C, D, E**

Midafternoon Snack: **A, B, C, D**

Dinner: **A, B, C, D, E**

PM Snack: **A, D**

GAZPACHO

5 to 6 ripe tomatoes, seeded and quartered
1 cucumber, peeled and seeded
½ onion, chopped
½ green pepper, chopped
¼ cup fresh cilantro, chopped
2 tbsp. chopped fresh basil or 1 tbsp. dried
1 tbsp. vinegar
3 cloves garlic, minced
Juice of ½ lemon
2 tbsp. chopped fresh parsley
½ tsp. dried oregano

Place the tomatoes, cucumber, onion, and green pepper in a blender and process until liquefied. Add the remaining ingredients and process again. If the mixture is too thick, add a few tablespoons of water or more lemon juice. If you like it spicier, add more seasonings to taste. Chill and serve cold. Makes 2 to 3 servings.

Compatible with Body Types:
Breakfast: N/A
Midmorning Snack: **A, B, C, D, E**
Lunch: **A, B, C, D, E**
Midafternoon Snack: **A, B, C, D**
Dinner: **A, B, C, D, E**
PM Snack: **A, D**

SUMMER SQUASH MEDLEY

3 to 4 zucchini, sliced
1 yellow or crookneck squash, sliced
5 to 6 pattypan squash, sliced or halved
½ onion, sliced
1 red pepper, chopped

Combine the squash, onion, and pepper in a vegetable steamer. Steam for about 5 minutes or until the vegetables are tender. These varieties of squash will cook quickly. If you overcook them, they will be mushy and lose their flavor. Makes 4 servings.

Compatible with Body Types:
Breakfast: N/A
Midmorning Snack: **A, B, C, D, E**
Lunch: **A, B, C, D, E**
Midafternoon Snack: **A, B, C, D**
Dinner: **A, B, C, D, E**
PM Snack: **A, D**

SPICY ASPARAGUS

1 cup fresh asparagus
1 cup pearl onions, peeled
½ cup finely chopped celery
1 tbsp. balsamic vinegar
¼ tsp. dill seed
¼ tsp. cayenne pepper
Black pepper, freshly ground, to taste

Steam the asparagus until it is almost completely cooked. Place it in a non-stick skillet and add the remaining ingredients, mixing well. Cover and cook over medium-high heat until the asparagus and pearl onions finish cooking, stirring often. Makes 2 servings.

Compatible with Body Types:
    Breakfast: N/A
    Midmorning Snack: **A, B, C, D, E**
    Lunch: **A, B, C, D, E**
    Midafternoon Snack: **A, B, C, D**
    Dinner: **A, B, C, D, E**
    PM Snack: **A, D**

OVEN-BAKED FRENCH FRIES

    2 baking potatoes
    1 sweet potato
    1 egg white
    ½ tsp. ground red pepper
    1 tbsp. chili powder
    ½ tsp. Mrs. Dash

Preheat the oven to 450 degrees. Cut the potatoes and sweet potato into thin fries. In a large bowl, lightly beat the egg white with a fork until foamy. Stir in the spices. Add the potatoes and toss to coat well. Using a nonstick cooking sheet, spread the potatoes in a single layer. Bake for 30 to 35 minutes or until the potatoes are crisp and brown. Makes 3 to 6 servings (depending on meal plan).

Compatible with Body Types:
    Breakfast: N/A
    Midmorning Snack: N/A
    Lunch: **A**
    Midafternoon Snack: N/A
    Dinner: **A**
    PM Snack: N/A

OVEN POTATO CHIPS

Preheat the oven to 450 degrees. Use a nonstick cookie sheet or a cookie sheet sprayed with nonstick spray. Scrub potatoes and slice very thin. Place potato slices, one layer thick only, onto the cookie sheet. Sprinkle with garlic powder and paprika. If you like spicier chips, add some chili powder. Bake about 5 minutes, then turn the potatoes and cook until crisp. Estimate 1 potato or ½ potato per person (depending on meal plan).

Compatible with Body Types:
    Breakfast: N/A
    Midmorning Snack: N/A
    Lunch: **A**
    Midafternoon Snack: N/A
    Dinner: **A**
    PM Snack: N/A

PERFECT MASHED POTATOES

Bake potatoes at 400 degrees for 1 hour. While the potatoes are baking, wrap some unpeeled garlic cloves or small onions in foil (1 or 2 per potato) and roast with the potatoes in the oven. When the potatoes are done, slice them in half and scoop out the flesh. Mash with a fork or potato masher. Squeeze the garlic cloves or onions out of their skins and mash with the potatoes. Beat the potatoes. For liquid, add a small amount of water, Vegetable Broth (page 204), or fat-free chicken broth. Add some freshly ground black pepper. Serve as is or garnish with snipped chives or minced parsley. Estimate 1 potato or ½ potato per person (depending on meal plan).

Compatible with Body Types:
    Breakfast: N/A
    Midmorning Snack: N/A
    Lunch: **A**
    Midafternoon Snack: N/A
    Dinner: **A**
    PM Snack: N/A

SPANISH RICE

    3 tbsp. tomato paste, sodium-free
    2 cups water
    1 cup rice
    ½ cup chopped onion
    ½ cup chopped green pepper
    2 tbsp. chopped fresh cilantro or parsley, or 1 tbsp. dried
    Chili powder (*optional*)

In a pot, mix the tomato paste with the water. Add the rice, onion, green pepper, cilantro or parsley, chili powder, and tomato paste and bring to a boil. After the water boils, turn the heat down to low and simmer for 20 to 30 minutes, or until all the water is absorbed. One cup of uncooked rice will yield 3 cups of cooked rice. This amount will yield six ½-cup servings.

Compatible with Body Types:

    Breakfast: N/A

    Midmorning Snack: N/A

    Lunch: **B, C, D, E**

    Midafternoon Snack: N/A

    Dinner: **B, C, D, E**

    PM Snack: N/A

WILD MUSHROOM AND TOMATO RICE

2 oz. crimini mushrooms, chopped

2 oz. portobello mushrooms, chopped

1 medium onion, chopped

1 green pepper, seeded and chopped

½ tsp. dried oregano

¼ to ½ tsp. freshly ground black pepper

1 cup uncooked rice

3 tomatoes, finely diced

½ cup red cooking wine

Place the mushrooms, onion, and green pepper in a nonstick skillet. Sauté over medium heat with 1 or 2 teaspoons of water until the onion is soft and translucent. Add the spices and rice and stir well for 1 minute. Add the tomatoes and wine. Bring to a boil, reduce the heat, cover, and cook for 30 minutes or until the rice is tender and the liquid is absorbed. One cup of uncooked rice will yield 3 cups of cooked rice. This amount will yield six ½-cup servings.

Compatible with Body Types:

    Breakfast: N/A

    Midmorning Snack: N/A

    Lunch: **B, C, D, E**

Midafternoon Snack: N/A
Dinner: **B, C, D, E**
PM Snack: N/A

CUCUMBER VINAIGRETTE

Try this recipe on a baked potato, as a salad dressing, or on fish or chicken. Peel, seed, and slice 1 cucumber. Process in the blender with a few drops of vinegar or lemon juice and a sprig of fresh dill and/or parsley. Add some mustard powder or Dijon mustard (sodium-free) and a dash of ground pepper. Blend until smooth. Chill and store in the refrigerator.

Compatible with Body Types:
Breakfast: N/A
Midmorning Snack: **A, B, C, D, E**
Lunch: **A, B, C, D, E**
Midafternoon Snack: **A, B, C, D, E**
Dinner: **A, B, C, D, E**
PM Snack: **A, D, E**

COLORFUL CABBAGE SLAW

4 cups shredded green cabbage
3 cups shredded red cabbage
½ cup thinly sliced green onions
1 red bell pepper, seeded and diced
½ cup apple cider vinegar
5 packages sugar substitute (such as Splenda or Equal), or to taste
1 tsp. freshly ground black pepper

oss the green and red cabbage, onion, and bell pepper in a large bowl. Mix the vinegar, sweetener, and black pepper in a separate bowl. Add the dressing to the cabbage mixture and mix well. Refrigerate several hours prior to serving. Makes seven 1-cup servings.

Compatible with Body Types:
 Breakfast: N/A
 Midmorning Snack: **A, B, C, D, E**
 Lunch: **A, B, C, D, E**
 Midafternoon Snack: **A, B, C, D, E**
 Dinner: **A, B, C, D, E**
 PM Snack: **A, D**

MEXICAN SALAD

 1 red onion, sliced
 1 bunch radishes
 2 tbsp. chopped fresh parsley
 5 to 6 ripe tomatoes, quartered
 1 cucumber, peeled and chopped
 ¼ cup fresh cilantro, chopped
 ½ tsp. black pepper
 Juice of 3 limes

Combine all the ingredients except the lime juice in a bowl. Add the lime juice and toss. Chill for an hour or two before serving. This has a wonderful flavor and will keep about 3 days in the refrigerator. Serve with chicken or fish. Makes five 1-cup servings.

Compatible with Body Types:
    Breakfast: N/A
    Midmorning Snack: **A, B, C, D, E**
    Lunch: **A, B, C, D, E**
    Midafternoon Snack: **A, B, C, D, E**
    Dinner: **A, B, C, D, E**
    PM Snack: **A, D**

CUCUMBER SALAD

    2 Japanese cucumbers, peeled
    ½ cup rice vinegar
    2 tsp. sugar substitute (such as Splenda or Equal)
    Dash of fresh or dried ginger
    Dash of red pepper flakes
    1 tsp. sesame seeds
    8 lettuce leaves

Slice the cucumbers paper-thin. Japanese cucumbers are the best, but regular can also be used; you may want to seed these. Combine the vinegar, sugar substitute, ginger, red pepper flakes, and sesame seeds in a bowl. This tastes best when prepared and allowed to stand overnight in the refrigerator. Serve on lettuce leaves. Makes 2 servings.

Compatible with Body Types:
    Breakfast: N/A
    Midmorning Snack: **A, B, C, D, E**
    Lunch: **A, B, C, D, E**
    Midafternoon Snack: **A, B, C, D, E**
    Dinner: **A, B, C, D, E**
    PM Snack: **A, D**

GREEN BEAN SALAD

1 lb. green beans, cut in 1-inch lengths
1 red pepper, seeded and chopped
1 yellow pepper, seeded and chopped
1 onion, chopped
1 clove garlic, minced or pressed
½ cup fresh parsley, chopped
Juice of 1 lemon
1 tbsp. vinegar
1 tsp. dry Dijon mustard (no salt added)
Freshly ground pepper

Steam the green beans for 8 to 10 minutes. Drain and combine with the red and yellow peppers, onion, garlic, and parsley. Combine the lemon juice, vinegar, and mustard. Toss with the beans, adding pepper to taste. Serve warm or chilled. Makes 4 servings.

Compatible with Body Types:
  Breakfast: N/A
  Midmorning Snack: **A, B, C, D, E**
  Lunch: **A, B, C, D, E**
  Midafternoon Snack: **A, B, C, D, E**
  Dinner: **A, B, C, D, E**
  PM Snack: **A, D**

Tips for Cooking Fresh Vegetables

ASPARAGUS

Asparagus spears are best when steamed for a brief period so that they maintain a slightly crisp texture when eaten. If steamed longer, they tend to get mushy. Be sure to cut off the tough ends at the bottom prior to steaming. Wash the asparagus, then steam for 5 to 7 minutes. Serve with a squeeze of fresh lemon and a dash of freshly grated black pepper.

BROCCOLI

Wash the broccoli. Cut off any tough ends. Peel the stems if they are quite thick or tough. Steam for 12 to 15 minutes, or until it is cooked the way you like it (from crisp to more soft). Steamed broccoli tastes delicious when served with freshly squeezed lemon juice and some freshly grated pepper.

BRUSSELS SPROUTS

If you have only eaten these frozen, you're in for a treat when you try them fresh. They are quite flavorful. Wash, trim the leaves, and cut off the stems. Steam for 12 to 15 minutes. Serve with freshly squeezed lemon juice, or season with freshly grated gingerroot, fresh garlic, and lemon.

CABBAGE

You can shred or chop a head of cabbage, or cut it into wedges, then steam or stir-fry it with other vegetables. A good shortcut if you're busy is to buy packages of preshredded cabbage for coleslaw. It will steam or stir-fry quickly. Try seasoning it with fresh parsley or cilantro, dill, or a little ginger.

CAULIFLOWER

A member of the cabbage family, cauliflower can be cooked much like broccoli. Wash, trim the outer leaves, and remove any tough ends of the stem. Steam for 10 to 12 minutes. Like brussels sprouts, steamed cauliflower tastes delicious with freshly squeezed lemon juice.

CELERY

Celery is a wonderful accompaniment to other vegetables such as cabbage, onions, and mushrooms in a stir-fry. Or you might try adding chopped celery to chopped carrots and onions and steaming all these veggies together.

MIXED VEGETABLES

For variety and great flavor, I suggest that you cook vegetables in combos. Here are some combinations, including suggestions for stir-frying your vegetables, that not only taste delicious but are very filling as well:

Asparagus and mushrooms
Broccoli and cauliflower
Eggplant, zucchini, mushrooms, and onions
Okra, tomatoes, green peppers, and onions
Red, yellow, and green peppers with mushrooms and onions
Spinach and mushrooms
Spinach and scallions with garlic
Spinach, tomatoes, and garlic
Tomatoes, cucumbers, radishes, and green onions
Zucchini, red peppers, and mushrooms

MUSHROOMS

Mushrooms have their own unique, subtle flavor and taste delicious by themselves or with other vegetables. Steam or stir-fry mushrooms. Mushrooms also make a delightful seasoning. You can cook them with chicken to add a subtle flavor. An easy, delicious dish is to sauté chicken breasts with mushrooms, onion, and some garlic. For variety, try some of the more exotic types of mushrooms that are now available in the produce section of grocery stores.

STIR-FRY VEGETABLE COMBINATIONS

Asparagus, celery, mushrooms, and onions
Bok choy, onions, mushrooms, chopped broccoli, and celery
Shredded cabbage, pea pods, chopped broccoli, and celery
Shredded broccoli, red peppers, and mushrooms
Shredded cabbage, onions, and celery

Desserts

STRAWBERRY DELIGHT

> 4 cups strawberries, halved
> 1 tbsp. sugar substitute (such as Splenda)
> 1 tbsp. golden balsamic vinegar

Clean and prepare the strawberries. Place the berries in a container. Mix the Splenda and balsamic vinegar and pour over the berries. Toss well. Place the container in the refrigerator and let stand for at least 30 minutes. Toss well before serving. Makes 4 to 8 servings (depending on meal plan).

Compatible with Body Types:
Breakfast: **A, B, C**
Midmorning Snack: N/A
Lunch: N/A
Midafternoon Snack: N/A
Dinner: N/A
PM Snack: **B, C, D**

FRUITY CUSTARD

> 4 egg whites
> 1 cup berries, lightly mashed
> ⅛ tsp. vanilla extract
> Sugar substitute (such as Splenda) to taste, if desired
> Dash of cinnamon
> Dash of nutmeg

Preheat the oven to 300 degrees. Combine all the ingredients in mixing bowl and beat until well mixed but not too frothy. Pour equally into 2 custard cups.

Set into a pan with ¾ inch of water in the bottom and bake for 30 to 45 minutes or until set (a knife inserted in the center will come out clean). Remove from the oven, cool, and refrigerate before serving. Makes 1 to 2 servings (depending on meal plan).

Compatible with Body Types:
    Breakfast: **B, C**
    Midmorning Snack: N/A
    Lunch: N/A
    Midafternoon Snack: N/A
    Dinner: N/A
    PM Snack: N/A

FRUIT SHAKE

1 lemon
2 packages sugar substitute (such as Splenda or Equal)
4 cups ice
Your portion of fruit, such as ½ cup strawberries
½ cup water

Squeeze the juice from the lemon, and pour the juice into a blender. Add the sweetener, fruit, and 2 cups of the ice. Blend to your desired consistency. Add in last 2 cups of ice and water. Stir to mix (in the blender), then blend again. Makes 1 serving.

Compatible with Body Types:
    Breakfast: **B, C**
    Midmorning Snack: N/A
    Lunch: N/A
    Midafternoon Snack: N/A
    Dinner: N/A
    PM Snack: N/A

EGG WHITE MERINGUE COOKIES

3 to 4 egg whites at room temperature
1 tbsp. apple cider vinegar
½ cup sugar substitute (such as Splenda or Equal)
1 tsp. vanilla extract

Preheat the oven to 300 degrees. Place the egg whites in a mixing bowl along with the vinegar. Start mixing on high speed until you can see that soft peaks are starting to form. Continue beating, slowly adding in the vanilla and sugar substitute. Once you have added those ingredients, be prepared to beat for a while— at least 8 to 10 minutes, until the peaks are stiff. Use a piece of parchment paper on your cookie sheets, and spoon out tablespoon-sized dollops. Bake for 30 to 40 minutes, until the cookies are lightly brown on top. Makes 1 serving.

Compatible with Body Types:
Breakfast: **B, C, D, E**
Midmorning Snack: N/A
Lunch: N/A
Midafternoon Snack: N/A
Dinner: N/A
PM Snack: N/A

BROILED CINNAMON GRAPEFRUIT

1 grapefruit
Dash of cinnamon
1 packet sugar substitute (such as Splenda or Equal)

Peel the grapefruit and take the skin off each section. Mix the grapefruit with cinnamon and Splenda. Eat cold or, if desired, broil until the Splenda caramelizes. Makes 1 serving (depending on meal plan).

Compatible with Body Types:
    Breakfast: **A, B, C**
    Midmorning Snack: N/A
    Lunch: N/A
    Midafternoon Snack: N/A
    Dinner: N/A
    PM Snack: **B, C, E**

RICE PUDDING

    1 tbsp. unsweetened applesauce
    ½ or 1 cup leftover rice
    1 egg white
    ½ tsp. cinnamon
    ½ tsp. vanilla extract
    Sugar substitute (such as Splenda or Equal), to taste

Add the applesauce to the leftover rice. Beat in the egg white. Add the cinnamon, vanilla extract, and sugar substitute. Microwave until the egg white is fully cooked. Makes 1 serving.

Compatible with Body Types:
    Breakfast: N/A
    Midmorning Snack: N/A
    Lunch: **B, C, D, E**
    Midafternoon Snack: N/A
    Dinner: **B, C, D, E**
    PM Snack: N/A

Customizations for Special Medical Conditions

Many of you may face special challenges when it comes to losing weight and following a specific eating plan. Please read this section carefully if you have hypoglycemia, diabetes, blood pressure problems, a thyroid condition, digestive disorders, or high cholesterol; if you are taking medication; or if you suffer from any type of medical condition. Do your Blueprint and select your custom eating plan, but before beginning, be sure to show this plan to your physician and have him or her make any additional customizations for you. I always advise my clients to *take their makeover program to their doctors* so that they can be fully informed about the diet and exercise issues involved. All my makeover programs, including the *6-Day Body Makeover,* are designed for men and women in normal health to help them lose weight and become even healthier in the process. Anyone who has a diagnosed medical condition, women who are pregnant or lactating, and women who are thinking about becoming pregnant, should not go on this program or any other reducing program until they have approval from their physician.

Hypoglycemia (Low Blood Sugar)

Hypoglycemia is a very pronounced reaction to diet, missed meals, and vigorous physical activity in which your blood sugar (glucose) falls sharply. When insufficient glucose in the blood is circulating in your nervous system and other cells, they become energy-starved. Some common symptoms include:

- Weakness

- Trembling

- Shakiness

- Dizziness

- Inability to concentrate

- Quick outbreak of perspiration

- Blurred vision

- Fainting (in extreme cases)

If you experience any of these symptoms after just an hour or two without food, chances are you have hypoglycemia, and you should consult your doctor prior to beginning this program.

Hypoglycemia can also cause you to misjudge your hunger. Low glucose levels can make you feel ravenous, and you will reach for anything and everything to remedy the low. At that point, it can be hard to control what you eat, and it becomes too easy to binge yourself right off your eating plan.

Generally, if you're eating at scheduled times on your custom eating plan, your blood sugar should stay relatively even. But if you still find yourself suffering from low blood sugar, you'll want to tweak your plan to avoid the disturbing symptoms of glucose depletion. In the chart on page 225 are some solutions to help you.

Should you wind up in an emergency situation, you'll need to get a simple sugar into your body as quickly as possible. Fruit juice, dried fruits, oranges, or even several jelly beans will help alleviate the symptoms. Waiting too long before eating can be danger-

Body Type A   Adjust your eating plan to include an extra carbohydrate at breakfast. This carbohydrate may be a potato or yam (in your designated serving size); an additional serving of grapefruit or berries; or 1 cup of cooked oatmeal (men) or ½ cup of cooked oatmeal (women). To keep your blood sugar at safe levels, do not skip any meals.

Body Type B   Adjust your eating plan to include an extra carbohydrate at breakfast. This carbohydrate may be rice (in your designated serving size) or an additional serving of grapefruit or berries. To keep your blood sugar at safe levels, do not skip any meals.

Body Type C   Adjust your eating plan to include an extra carbohydrate at breakfast. This carbohydrate may be rice (in your designated serving size) or an additional serving of grapefruit or berries. To keep your blood sugar at safe levels, do not skip any meals.

Body Type D   Adjust your eating plan to include a carbohydrate at breakfast. This carbohydrate may be rice (in your designated serving size). To keep your blood sugar at safe levels, do not skip any meals.

Body Type E   Adjust your eating plan to include a carbohydrate at breakfast. This carbohydrate may be rice or rice and beans (in your designated serving size), or a serving of grapefruit or berries. To keep your blood sugar at safe levels, do not skip any meals.

ous. You could faint or go into shock. The longer you wait, the more difficult it is to bring your blood sugar back in balance.

If you are inclined toward hypoglycemia, be prepared for emergencies. One solution is to carry raisins or a Clif Bar with you at all times. A tablespoon of raisins will short-circuit the onset of hypoglycemic symptoms. If your symptoms are severe, eat pie, ice cream, or another high-sugar food. But as soon as you can, consume a slow carbohydrate, which converts to sugar in the body more gradually, along with some protein. This combination of foods leads to a more even blood sugar level and more sustained energy. Never eat protein by itself; this will drive your blood sugar even lower.

Most of us will experience low blood sugar at some point or another, so it's important to know the symptoms and how to handle them. If you are extremely hypoglycemic, however, you may need to add a carbohydrate to every one of your meals. Make sure your physician helps you customize your diet.

High Blood Pressure (Hypertension)

Largely a symptomless disease, high blood pressure affects one in four Americans. Normal blood pressure is equal to or less than 120 over 80 most of the time. The top number refers to systolic pressure, the pressure in the artery when the heart contracts; the lower number refers to diastolic pressure, the pressure in the artery when the heart relaxes. Every incremental hike in blood pressure corresponds to a rise in your risk of heart attack, heart failure, stroke, and kidney disease.

If you have been diagnosed with high blood pressure, your custom eating plan will help you considerably, since it is very low in sodium, one of the chief instigators of high blood pressure. Low-sodium diets do a lot to nudge your blood pressure down, and every little bit of pressure lowering helps. Losing weight also helps get your blood pressure back into the safety zone.

With high blood pressure, however, you may want to eliminate egg whites (if your eating plan calls for them), which are very high in sodium. You may substitute another source of protein for the egg whites, such as fish or lean poultry. Diets that are well populated with fish somehow seem to counteract high blood pressure.

Also, make sure you review your eating plan with your doctor, particularly if you are taking blood pressure medication. Even after following your eating plan for just six days, your blood pressure may drop naturally, and your doctor may then need to adjust your medication accordingly.

Low Blood Pressure (Hypotension)

As I mentioned above, normal blood pressure is 120/80 or lower. Unlike high blood pressure, there are no clear-cut standards for the diagnosis of low blood pressure. If your doctor says your blood pressure is unusually low, this should be evaluated medically, since low blood pressure isn't a specific disease but rather the sign of some underlying medical problem. There are telltale symptoms of low blood pressure, however, and these include:

- Tiredness
- Weakness
- Headaches
- Heart palpitations
- Fainting
- Dizziness

With low blood pressure, you need some sodium in your diet. That being the case, add a little salt to your diet, particularly in the morning. No-sodium-added canned tuna and low-sodium soy sauce are two excellent ways to incorporate some sodium into your diet without triggering too much water retention. If you suffer from symptoms of low blood pressure, try to have a source of salt on hand at all times. Carrying a few salt packets in your pocket is a good solution. Consume one right away if you start to feel dizzy or light-headed. One of the best moves you can make is to add salt to a beverage such as Gatorade in order to elevate your blood pressure to more normal levels. In addition, make sure your doctor reviews your customized eating plan.

Diabetes

A sugar metabolism disorder, diabetes is a serious, potentially life-threatening disease. Even though the *6-Day Body Makeover* eating plans can help regulate blood sugar in people with diabetes, you should not begin this program without consulting your doctor first, particularly if you are insulin-dependent.

If you are overweight and have type 2 diabetes (also called non-insulin-dependent diabetes mellitus, or NIDDM), weight loss through diet and regular exercise can be essential to controlling the disease. In many cases, losing weight makes it possible for people with type 2 diabetes to discontinue taking medication for diabetes altogether. Weight loss may also reduce cholesterol and blood pressure, both of which are commonly elevated in this form of the disease.

Because your custom eating plan, in conjunction with diabetes medications, may lower your blood sugar, it is important to carry glucose tablets with you in case you suffer an emergency bout with hypoglycemia.

Ulcers and Other Digestive Disorders

Digestive troubles plague millions of Americans and can be made worse by offending foods. With problems such as ulcers, you'll want to identify foods that aggravate the problem, then correct your course nutritionally, under the guidance of your physician. Here are a few general pointers:

- Avoid raw vegetables.
- Cook your vegetables to help break them down and make it easier for your body to digest.
- Eat whipped or mashed potatoes, if your eating plan prescribes them.
- Avoid salt and spices.
- Eat very light fish (such as sole or flounder), ground turkey breast, and egg whites, where your eating plan calls for these foods.

If you suffer from inflammatory bowel disease (IBD) such as Crohn's disease, or ulcerative colitis or other digestive disorders such as diverticulosis or spastic colon, always consult your physician before changing your diet.

Thyroid Disease

Straddling your windpipe is a bow-tie-shaped mass of tissue called the thyroid gland. It produces specific hormones that set your metabolic tempo. If that tempo is slow—a condition called hypothyroidism or underactive thyroid—your thyroid gland may not be producing enough hormones, and your body's food-handling ability is compromised. Instead of being converted into energy, food is mostly stockpiled as body fat.

If you are eating according to your plan and still find you have trouble losing weight, it may be a good idea to see your physician and request a thyroid function test. This test checks your blood for levels of thyroid hormones to determine whether these levels are within a normal range. If you are diagnosed with an underactive thyroid, it can be treated and corrected with prescription thyroid medication.

Pregnant or Nursing

Do not follow the *6-Day Body Makeover* if you are pregnant or nursing. Your body requires extra calories at this time. Save this program until you've stopped nursing. It is a great tool for shedding postpregnancy pounds in a hurry.

Menopause

Many women still take estrogen in the form of birth control pills or hormone replacement therapy (although estrogen therapy is prescribed less and less for women undergoing menopause). Unfortunately, estrogen directly affects weight gain, including where fat is deposited (including breasts, buttocks, hips, and thighs). It also promotes water retention. This does not mean, however, that you cannot lose weight. It just means that you may lose it more slowly, in general. Some good news, though: The *6-Day Body Makeover* has proven to be an effective tool for women in menopause who need to kick-start their fat-burning mechanisms, despite taking supplemental estrogen.

Food Allergies

Food allergies can be a hidden cause of weight gain, and the "usual suspects" provoking reactions in susceptible people are milk, eggs, peanuts, soy foods, wheat, fish, and shellfish. If you know you're allergic to certain foods, don't eat them! Working with your physician, identify alternatives that you can tolerate.

High Cholesterol

If you have high cholesterol, avoid red meat and shellfish, regardless of what body type you have. The saturated fat and dietary cholesterol in these foods contribute to high cholesterol in the blood, which in turn clogs blood vessels and increases your risk of heart attack and stroke. For protein, stick with lean poultry and fish instead. Finally, make sure you review your eating plan with your doctor.

Dry Skin or Hair

If your skin or hair is unusually dry, add a little more fat to your diet. There are ways to do this without destroying your fat loss. For example, add about a teaspoon of flaxseed oil to your salad. Or you can substitute a fattier fish such as salmon, trout, or sea bass for one of your proteins. If you do this, eliminate the carbohydrate at that meal and substitute extra greens instead. Here's why: Additional fat taken with carbohydrates has the unfortunate consequence of being more readily stored. Eliminating the carb will prevent this from happening and keep your weight loss on target. Plus, the fat in the fish or flaxseed oil helps sustain your glucose levels so that your blood sugar doesn't plummet too much from lack of carbs. Obviously, be extremely cautious about this sort of dietary manipulation if you are prone to hypoglycemia.

On Any Medication

You may be surprised to learn that there are more than 100 prescription medications with the common side effect of weight gain. Some of the worst offenders are antidepressants, blood pressure drugs, steroids, diabetic medicines, hormone replacement therapy, and anti-seizure medications. If you are taking any of these drugs or others, talk to your doctor about whether they may interfere with your desire to lose weight. Never discontinue taking a drug or adjusting your dosage without first consulting with your doctor.

In addition, some drugs interact adversely with medications (grapefruit and grapefruit juice are two examples), so make sure your physician is familiar with your eating plan and can review it before you start your body makeover.

Additional Resources

Food and Nutrition Information

For nutritional information on various foods, log on to CalorieKing.com, a searchable database of more than 30,000 generic and brand-name foods, including more than 150 fast-food chains.

Continuum Health Partners, Inc., features a fiber content chart at http://www.we healny.org/healthinfo/dietaryfiber/fibercontentchart.html. The foods are organized by fiber and calorie content; the list includes foods with no fiber.

Resistance Training

American College of Sports Medicine (ACSM): Log on to www.acsm.org for information on resistance training, working out at home or at an exercise facility, selecting a personal trainer, and more. The ACSM advances and integrates scientific research to provide educational and practical applications of exercise science and sports medicine.

National Strength and Conditioning Association (NSCA): For help in finding an NSCA-certified personal trainer, log on to www.nsca-lift.org. The NSCA also has online articles covering all aspects of strength and conditioning.

Information on Medical Conditions

If you suffer from any of the conditions listed in appendix B, learn more about your treatment options by logging on to www.webMD.com. WebMD provides valuable health information, tools for managing your health, and support to those who seek information.

Michael Thurmond's Makeover Programs

Log on to www.provida.com for information on additional tools you need to make over your body and stay motivated. There is also information on my Living Lean maintenance program so that you can keep your body at your goal weight.

When you have a question about any aspect of my programs, you can get the answer you need, on the phone or online, from one of my specially trained *6-Week Body Makeover* specialists. This assistance is available 24 hours a day and includes a recipe database, success stories, nutritional research updates, and other information.

Also available 24 hours a day is an online support community. In this supportive forum, you can ask questions, get answers, share stories, and get motivated.

Additional information is available at www.bodymakeover.com.

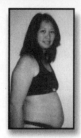 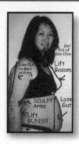 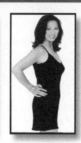
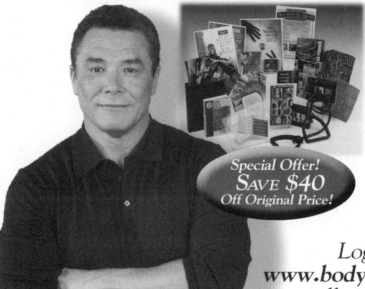